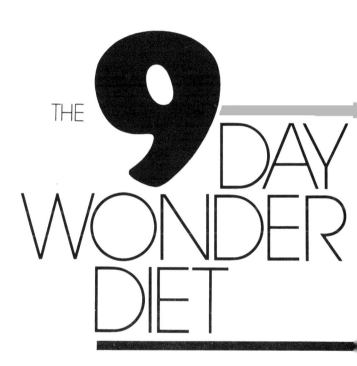

THE **9** DAY
WONDER
DIET

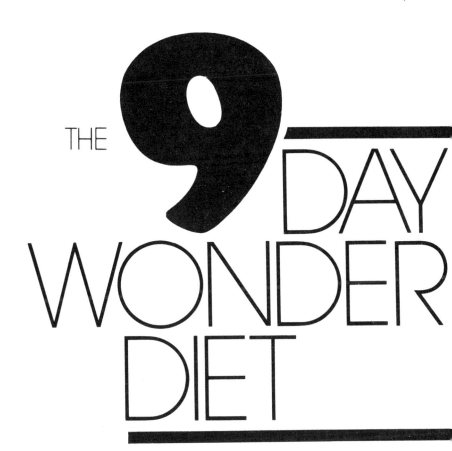

THE **9** DAY WONDER DIET

Dr. Seymour Isenberg
Dr. L. M. Elting

St. Martin's Press
New York

For Tiffany
who wanted her breakfast

Copyright © 1978 by Seymour Isenberg and L. Melvin Elting
All rights reserved. For information, write:
St. Martin's Press, Inc., 175 Fifth Ave., New York, N.Y. 10010.
Manufactured in the United States of America

Library of Congress Cataloging in Publication Data

Isenberg, Seymour.
    The nine day wonder diet.

    1. Reducing diets.   2. Reducing exercises.
I. Elting, Melvin, joint author.   II. Title.
RM222.2.I83   613.2′5   77-16738

ISBN 0-312-57391-X

Portions of the first chapter of this book were excerpted
in Cosmopolitan's *Super Diets And Exercise Guide.*

CONTENTS

the Weekend...The Cyclical Nature of the Plan...Why We Devised the Nine-Day Plan...Why You Can Lose Weight This Way Even If You're a Three- or Four-Time Loser...Why It Is Safe and Healthy to Lose Weight This Way...Hidden Calories...Salt...What About Alcohol?...Using Food Itself to Control Your Weight...Water Is a Must...Your CBO (Calorie Burn-Out) Time... Empty Calories and Full Calories...Sauces and Cheeses...Eggs and Fowl...Some Supplemental Backups...Multi-vitamin-mineral Supplements...Methylcellulose...Bran Tablets...Protein Hydrosolate Liquid...If You Get Sick...Spot Reducing...How the Nine-Day Plan Reduces Those Troublesome Areas...You, Too, Can Be a Success

Nausea...Constipation...Fatigue...Exercise
...Work...Feeling Cold...Feeling Warm...Tension...The People Around You...Extra Added
Benefits...Sex and Fasting...Fasting Gives Your
Body a Rest...What Happens to Hunger?...The
"Total Contentment" Pill...The Must Items for
This Day...Morning...Afternoon...Evening...
If You Can't Fast All Day...Partial Fasting: List
#1 (dinner only)...Partial Fasting: List #2
(lunch only)...If You Require Lunch and Dinner...Partial Fasting: List #3 (breakfast only)
...Combining Breakfast with Lunch and Dinner

7 DAY 4: TUESDAY: THE SECOND FAST DAY

You're Doing It Easier...More Energy Today
...Relaxing Tension...The Must Items for
This Day...Instructions for the Day...Breaking the Fast...Fast Breaking Menu...If
You Can't Fast on the 2nd Day...Partial Fasting: List #1 (dinner only)...Snacking in
Place of Dinner...Partial Fasting: List #2
(lunch only)...Today's Lunch-Dinner Combination...Partial Fasting: List #3 (breakfast
only)...Combining All Meals Today...and
If You've Fasted

8 DAY 5: WEDNESDAY: THE FULL PROTEIN DAY

Getting on the Scale...How You Will Eat Today
...What You Will Eat Today...Basic Menu for
Day 5...Today's Time Zones...Alternate
Menus to Today's Plan...Keep Cool...Recipes for
Alternate Menus...Act Like a Winner and
You'll be a Loser

Come what come may
Time and the hour runs through the roughest day.
Macbeth

AUTHORS' NOTE

We've organized both book and diet as a day by day process. Best results on this plan have been obtained by people who read and diet step by step, day by day. So rather than read the whole book first, familiarize yourself with the general introductory material and then start right in with Day One — each new day will hold surprises.

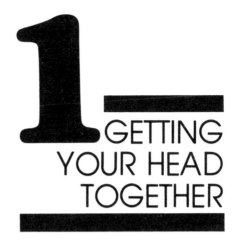

1
GETTING YOUR HEAD TOGETHER

Success in following any diet depends on your frame of mind. Sure, you've done it before; you know the dry taste of defeat. But if you look on your forthcoming plan as an ordeal, you will surely fail once again. On the other hand, your chances of making it to that slim, trim You that you want to be are enhanced by taking a positive attitude and working out some of the kinks ahead of time. Remember, no matter how you slice it, you're going to be slicing it thinner, divorcing yourself from some of your favorite treats and eating habits. As in any divorce, the more unprepared you are, the more difficult a time you will have.

Therefore, approach your diet as a provocative occasion. One good reason for attempting it is to increase your desirability as a sensual man or woman—to whet someone else's appetite by getting yours under control. Isn't it provocative to realize that the only thing standing between you and a truly fantastic sex life is a few pounds? Are you going to let them stand in your way?

No way!

So before getting into the basic plan, we'd like to make a few suggestions to start you off on the right foot.

1

STOP BUYING CLOTHES

Every time you buy more clothes to fit you at your present weight you compromise with it. "I feel sick about my weight," one thirty-year-old woman confided to us, "and the only way I feel better is to buy some new clothes. It takes my mind off food. It's either that or eat." In fact it was both. She was steadily getting heavier. You can't substitute putting something on your back for putting something in your mouth. The two are inseparable. Once you've bought those new clothes, cleverly tailored to disguise and flatter your figure, you'll actually *feel* thinner. You'll spend hours seeking out garments that will disguise the real you, and when your friends tell you how thin you look, how much convincing do you think you'll need to believe it? It's easy to put your faith in your own sartorial propaganda; unfortunately it leaves you as fat, if not fatter, than ever.

In addition, new clothes purchased for the Overweight You will give you an allegedly practical reason not to start on a diet. After all, once you start losing weight, these items won't fit you . . . you may as well wear them in a bit . . . you can supply all the other reasons that we fat people use to deceive ourselves.

In any event, the new clothes shortly won't fit you anyway, as the weight keeps going on.

Do just the opposite. As you lose weight, get rid of your "fat" clothes. Burning your Balenciagas and your Brooks Brothers behind you gives you a new sense of identity, a feeling that you've taken your destiny in your hands and are stepping forth to irreversible success.

ENTERTAIN MORE AT HOME

Going out is fun but it can be unnecessarily challenging to your self-control. Severe self-discipline will sooner or later only result in your eating those items you're supposed to be disciplining yourself against. So don't rely on your self-control—certainly not at the start. After all, if you had self-control, you wouldn't be in your present fix. And with everyone at the table eating all those fattening things with such abandon—and encouraging you to eat them as well—self-control goes right out the window.

2

In fact, self-control, like charity, begins at home. Now, don't misunderstand us. We're not saying you can't go out. We are saying that for the extent of your diet you should be prepared to pick and choose such occasions with care. For the most part, have people in. You'll find it is fun to learn how to utilize the foods you are allowed. You'll discover how to make and serve them in all sorts of different ways. Remember, too, that at your house you control the meals; you aren't at the mercy of some outside cook. And keep in mind that "going out" can also mean just a night at the local movie house. True, many people go to eat afterwards. If you are out with another couple, invite them for a bite back to your place, where you can control the situation. Don't end up using the movie as a springboard to clear your diet. You'll hate yourself in the morning, especially when you step on the scale.

KEEP IT OUT OF THE HOUSE

If it isn't on your diet, don't have it in your refrigerator. Forbidden tidbits, invested with a life of their own, seem to ooze in through the pores. If it isn't around, you can't eat it and, since most people do their eating at night, it is unlikely that you would run out to the supermarket to indulge your fancy at midnight. Convenience is one of the things that has gotten you fat; make it inconvenient to have such items on hand. If you're having a party, send the dessert home with the guests. If you're having another party next day, buy all new ingredients. The old ones wouldn't make it anyway—not with you in the house.

KEEP YOUR MOUTH SHUT ABOUT YOUR DIET

Opening your mouth has always gotten you into trouble; keep it closed. You have no friends when it comes to losing weight. All your friends are probably experts on the subject. Most people have attempted to lose weight at some time or other, and even if what they tried didn't work for them, they're sure it would be just the thing for you. This makes everyone an "authority."

There are your thin friends, who have no conception of *your* problem and will likely attempt to steer you off your plan at the first

¾-pound loss. "You'll make yourself sick," they'll cry with horror, thus giving you a great excuse to go back to eating.

If your friends are fat themselves, you may be even more inclined to share with them the new diet you are following. But your fat friends may not really *want* to lose weight. They aren't really willing to try, but they don't want you to lose, either. The thinner *you* get, the fatter *they* look. It's easier for them to keep you from losing than for them to lose. If you let them, they'll destroy all the confidence you've built up in your diet with their handy little negativisms.

How do you diet without telling anybody what you are doing? Make up the most bizarre excuse you can think of, as personal as possible. The more personal it is, the less people will tend to pursue it. Your weight should be a personal enough reason, but you will find that your weight seems to be everybody's business.

"It interferes with my sex life" is one excuse you can offer for why you're not eating something. "It makes me break out" is another. And, for you women, there's always that universal scapegoat, your period, to blame it on. Whatever excuse you use, don't laugh or joke when you offer it. Losing weight is a serious business, and if your friends or relatives are going to be on your back, you can only get heavier.

SET A REASONABLE GOAL

Of course you want to lose all your weight tomorrow. Who doesn't? Unfortunately, you won't. Not even the day after tomorrow. Studies have shown that most diets based on fact rather than fantasy can safely take off an average of two pounds a week. We're going to show you here how you can lose a lot more than that in slightly over a week—anywhere between eight to twelve pounds in nine days—but if you've a lot more than that to lose, your average loss recycling on this plan will be approximately two to three pounds per week. That's a loss of over seven thousand calories.

BUY A SPECIAL NOTEBOOK

You should keep some sort of record of your daily food intake as well as a diary of events relating to your instances of eating or not eating. This is much better than a vague reliance on memory, since

4

it will provide you with actual *specifics* tomorrow about what you did or did not accomplish today. In order to start off your new plan with a clean slate, you must first buy one. Don't settle for the ordinary notepaper you have on hand. That won't give you the effect of a brand-new attempt. Get hold of an inexpensive but efficient-looking record book, open it to the first page and begin a new chapter in your life. Writing down what you do will keep providing you with the knowledge that, notwithstanding how many diets you've tried in the past, with this one you are truly turning over a new leaf every day.

LIST YOUR EATING HABITS

Write down all the food you eat and the water and other liquids you consume each day. On those days that you do not eat, write down your impressions. You may get dizzy or have a temporary feeling of nausea. You may never have felt so good. Such notes are invaluable in comparing the different days of the cycle. If you feel dizzy one time, check back to see how you felt doing this identical thing before; if you find you weren't dizzy then, chances are that something other than your diet plan is causing it.

If you wish, you may total up the calories at the end of the day, but many diets do not call for this and we have never found it essential. What is important is writing everything down at the time you eat or drink it, or as close thereto as you can reasonably make it. We've often heard patients say, "I really starved myself yesterday." Yet these individuals, when their memory is jogged fairly intensively, quite often remember that they'd eaten things they hadn't really considered. They'd done it without thinking and then repressed it. One woman had gone through an entire can of nuts, three candy bars and half a pizza. However, what she recalled was that she'd carefully avoided eating breakfast, lunch or dinner; therefore she'd done pretty well. Silly, you think? Not a bit of it. Chances are, if you're honest about it, that you can remember having done the same thing yourself. The mind plays funny tricks, and you will find (if you haven't already) that where food is concerned, you're the craftiest person you know. So, in the endeavor to keep your head on straight, write down what you do with food.

5

Don't be ashamed of your habits; but recognize that you will either break them or they will break you. We want you to be proud of yourself—a pride based on an accurate appraisal of how you're handling your new weight-loss plan. Dieting involves being proud; why else would you put yourself through such a situation? And pride goeth before a fall...in weight.

In addition to listing the things you eat, be sure to list the time you eat, what room you eat in, what else you are doing during the eating process (such as reading, watching TV, arguing, and the like) and who else is present if you are not alone. You'll never really be alone because we'll be there with you through the pages of this book. We'll help you make a start and carry it through. But first you must understand some of the things that have helped get you fat. Studies have shown that only by understanding your eating pattern can you avoid getting back on it. So this book is meant not only to get you thin, but to keep you thin once you've lost your excess weight.

GET A GOOD SCALE

It's amazing to us how many people weigh themselves on obsolete devices, cheap scales they'd certainly balk at if an airline used them for weighing luggage. The whole idea of dieting is to obtain an accurate record of weight loss, not a guess. How else are you going to know how effective your plan is? Certainly if your scale is off you are going to be wasting a lot of time lying to yourself.

There are two ways to keep your scale in line. The first is to check it each time you use it. Since most people weigh themselves on the routine bathroom spring scale, which is easily affected by humidity, you must compensate for this. There are, of course, spring scales and spring scales. If you can afford it, get the top of the line. You didn't stint when it came to putting on the weight; don't stint now you're ready to take it off. You're going to need all the help you can get; have an accurate instrument that will honestly reflect your endeavors. However, even a good spring scale must be checked. Keep a known weight handy (a five-pound sack of flour will do) and make sure it weighs out to what it should. Take a few extra seconds rather than obtain a false report.

The other way to make certain of your true weight is not to use a scale at all, but a balance, similar to what you've seen in your doctor's office. This is a more expensive item than the bathroom scale and takes up a little more room, but it rarely has to be recalibrated and will last indefinitely. You are going to be giving it a lot of use; you will probably find it worth the investment.

WEIGH AND MEASURE YOURSELF

Your weight and inches should be recorded in your weight notebook. Weighing *always* should be done at the same time each day—that is, in the morning, upon arising and after urinating. It should always be done in the nude. If you miss the time, don't do it at all as your weight will not be accurate and you will dislocate all the data you've accumulated. You will also give your morale a blow it possibly will not survive. The temptation will always be there to get weighed at other times. We have patients who all but specialize in getting weighed... at friends' homes, on subway stations, bus platforms, at the local post office—anyplace they can find a scale. It can become addicting; you'll be weighing yourself until you get fed up—with the scale, not with eating—and that's a good way to go off any diet.

On this plan we do not suggest that you weigh yourself every day until you've completed the cycle. If you must know how you are doing before that, wait until at least the first four days have gone by. We don't know at which portion of the plan your weight loss will begin to show; our observations and patients' reports seem to indicate that loss on this plan is very individualistic, with some people showing a drop immediately, and others not until the very end of the cycle. But all told, we suggest that you don't check your weight more than three times during the cycle, including the final weighing at the end of the nine days.

What you must keep in mind is that just because your *psyche* has finally decided to lose doesn't mean that the rest of you will immediately cooperate. Give your body a chance to catch up with your determination. Don't lose the battle in rehearsal. You don't lose weight every day unless you have something very seriously wrong with you. Even at your most voracious, you didn't *gain* weight every day. It may have felt that way, but if that had indeed

7

been the case, you wouldn't be able to get through the doorway. You didn't rush home after gorging yourself at a wedding party and immediately jump on the scale to see how much you'd gained, did you? Few of us are quite that masochistic. Yet, if you had, chances are you would have been surprised to see that the weight gain was probably minimal. That doesn't mean you didn't do yourself damage, that you were able to eat and get away with it. No. All you did was move further along the scale to the next weight hike. For weight gain goes in increments: you gain and level off, gain and level off. These leveling-off areas are called plateaus. So, when you lose weight, your body accommodates itself to the same system in reverse. You lose and level off, lose and level off. And, so long as you follow your diet, even though your weight loss may not show on the scale, you are moving yourself along that plateau to the next weight-loss area. Where most people get discouraged is in not understanding this simple logic of the body. They look at the scale, see it has not registered a loss—and feel they've gone through all their work of dieting for nothing. There's no such thing as dieting for nothing; eventually, if the diet is one that is worthwhile, you will see results. Unfortunately, fat people are in a hurry. In this instance haste doesn't make waste, it makes more fat.

Measuring yourself is one way to see what is happening along the plateau area even if you don't have a weight loss. On this plan we recommend that you measure yourself three times: after the first three days, after the second three and, of course, at the end. Measure yourself in the following places, nude, with a seamstress' tape measure:

Breasts (across the nipple line)
Belly (across the belly button)
Hips (across the hip joint)
Thighs (halfway from knee to groin).

If you keep accurate measurements, you'll find yourself in a fascinating numbers game. You can lose inches and no weight, weight and no inches, both together or alternately. Taking measurements helps you realize what is happening inside your body, and the anatomic marks we have suggested you use are easy to find, so that you can always go back to the same places.

As your diet takes hold, your fat deposits begin to be mobilized as sugar—the ultimate energy requirement. This sugar is then taken from the fat and stored in the liver as liver sugar, or glycogen. From there it will go into the blood stream to be burned for energy. While in the liver it takes up less room than it did as fat—allowing you to lose inches—but it weighs exactly the same. Under these circumstances, were you to weigh yourself without measuring, you would assume that nothing was happening, get discouraged and go off your diet. In fact, that very day you gave up you would likely have lost weight. One very important thing to realize, therefore, is that the scale doesn't tell the whole story.

"I CAN'T EAT ALL THAT!"

One of the chief complaints we've run into about the first weekend is "too much food." One woman complained: "I really had to stuff myself. I can't eat all that."

We assure you, you needn't eat "all that." In fact, the less, the better. You may not lose weight faster—but you'll *feel* thinner. Don't let the scale discourage this feeling. The scale is always off as far as your inch loss is concerned. Even measuring yourself won't show the drop in inches as fast as it occurs because a portion of water is always left behind. The way you feel is far more accurate than any artificial measuring device; your internal barometer will tell you more surely than any mechanical instrument when you've lost—and when you've gained, even if the scale temporarily registers no change.

That's why we stress that you not depend on the scale, especially during the first weekend. You may find, weighing yourself at this time, that to your horror you actually weigh more. But bear in mind that your weight is still a reflection of your previous eating habits: your previous consumption of solids and fluids and, especially, of salt. But don't be concerned. Remember, you are on a Nine-Day Cycle, not a twenty-four- or forty-eight-hour one, and you have to give it a chance to take hold. This is not to say that it is to be expected that a weight gain will occur. The majority of people on the plan *did* experience some sort of loss after the first weekend, one lady dropping six pounds by Monday morning. But even here, the body tries to balance out. By the end of the cycle she had lost twelve pounds, not the twenty she had hoped for based on those first couple of days. Such is human nature that she was annoyed at the plan for not fulfilling the promise she had presumed into it. Don't be that way. Relax, do your job and your diet will take care of itself. Remember that every pound you lose is another that you didn't gain, so by the time you are through with your cycle, you've really lost twice as much as the scale shows.

GET YOUR PICTURE TAKEN

You don't like the idea? Of course not; most fat people don't. But this is for therapy, not vanity. We take pictures of all our patients—fully dressed—when we first meet with them and every twenty pounds thereafter. Now, you may not have twenty pounds to lose, but even the loss of ten pounds will make a decided difference in your body presentation to the camera; just this much weight loss will make your clothes hang differently and will significantly alter the way you stand. What you want is an image you can live up to, a new you that you can actually see and be proud of...as well as a warning, in the "before" picture, of the way things were when you were using the lower portion of your head more than the upper.

Have a friend take your picture, or do it yourself with a timer; an instant camera is probably most convenient. Take your repeat pictures at successive stages of weight loss depending on how far you have to go—say, every ten pounds. These pictures will do several things. First, they will show you that something is happening. You can't possibly remember bodily detail as well as a camera can. You will also be able to see where your weight is or is not coming off. Then there is the psychological therapy: each picture is another step forward, another hurdle from the girdle, a smaller size in suits, another light in the dieting darkness. Each picture closes an overweight door behind you.

Save your pictures. You'll need an image to stay thin by, and you'll forget what you looked like fat. This makes it all too easy to repeat the process. Many of our patients, comparing their present-weight pictures with their pre-diet ones will say, "Come on, I couldn't have looked like that." You looked like that.

HAVE A LOVE AFFAIR

You're married? Have an affair with your husband or wife. There's no reason to diet in this department. As your figure gets into shape, not only will you turn on, so will that certain someone. Lovemaking is not only a logical end result of losing weight because you look better, more sensuous—it actually helps the weight-loss process. Not from the standpoint of burning up calories, alas, since expenditure in this department is only about seventy calories per person—about the amount you'd lose briskly climbing a flight of stairs—but from the discovery that your lovemaking will be better than ever. That's enough of a stimulus to keep you on the most rigid diet, let alone one that is simple and easy. The emotional drive of sex also tends to have a dampening effect on the appetite center in the brain: the more attention you pay to sex; the less attention you will pay to food. (It works the other way as well: many obese people, interested mainly in food, have little interest in sex.)

So, you women, go out of your way to make yourself feel sexy, to look like the woman you know you can be. A new hairdo? Definitely. A pedicure? Of course. If you're not worth it, who is? While losing those excess pounds you must be sure not to neglect your basic femininity. Too many heavy women take a down attitude about themselves...won't use makeup, buy a new hat, have a permanent because "they aren't worth the trouble. I'm too grotesque." Yet how many ugly thin women take the trouble? Don't use your weight as a cop-out; work on your appearance to make yourself as provocative as possible. Intensify your sense of belonging to yourself. Strip yourself naked and look at yourself in the mirror. You can't hide any longer, you've no longer anything to be ashamed of, you're going to *succeed*. Some of the signs of your success may already be there in pounds and inches lost. You're on your way to another, thinner life and the time of hiding your head in the sand, your body behind a barrier of fabric to disguise it, is over. Take stock of yourself. Run your hands over your body, over the sides of your torso, over your waist. Which is it to be, waist or waste? The answer is obvious.

And you men, you're no different. Masculinity has never been portrayed as buried in fat. The girls have one over you here; some

11

of the greatest painters of the female figure, such as Rubens and Velasquez, preferred models at least thirty pounds over the norm and they still look perfectly delectable today. But in all artistic history, whether the medium be sculpture, painting or papier-mâché, the male figure is always portrayed as thin. It is up to you either to live up to or live down this artistic heritage. You've got a lot of good public relations going for you here; conversely, there's very little going for you fat. You, too, must learn to accept your body as your own, and something of value in its own right, not just think of it as something to feed and put clothes on. You like to think that women are vainer then men, and indeed, most of our patients are women. We don't think that makes them vainer—just smarter. And overweight is certainly not sexist; as many men suffer from the problem as do women. True, once they make up their minds to lose the weight, men are able, in many instances, to outdo the ladies in speed of removal. But that's only because they aren't subject to one week out of every month when their bodies retain fluid. And men make up for this more rapid loss by often becoming cocky, feeling they can continue to lose whenever they are so inclined, and ending up on a perpetual seesaw of weight loss-weight gain.

We say to you, as we said to the girls, become a more sensual individual by first recognizing that there is a problem, and then doing something about it...but don't wait until you are thin to begin enjoying your body. We don't want you to eat pie in the sky by and by. We want you to stop eating real pie now so as to enjoy the main course: a more effective you in every way.

EXERCISE

Right or wrong: Inside every fat person is a thin one trying to get out?

Wrong.

Outside every fat person is an even fatter one trying to get in.

That's the one that made you what you are today. That's the one to guard against—and rational exercise can help you do it. Let's face it, exercising really isn't fun. Mostly it is boring. And remember, running around doing housework or washing the car or walking the dog doesn't count as exercise in the way we mean it. To be effective, exercise must be something outside your daily routine that is done on a daily basis. It doesn't matter so much *what* exercise you do, it's *how often* you do it that counts. And its importance is not even so much for muscle tone (although that certainly improves) as for some of the physiologic changes that will occur. Your cholesterol levels, for instance, can be significantly lowered by exercising. That means you may well be less prone to a heart attack. Certain isometric exercises (certainly the safest form of exercise for fat people—they rely on muscle tensing rather than exertion) have been shown to lower high blood pressure safely. Such exercises can also dilate blood vessels that have been put into poor condition from smoking, and delay the aging process by improving your muscle tone. Remember, it is the skeletal muscles, those attached to the skeleton, that support your body and girdle in all those extra pounds. The tighter you make them, and that is really what is meant by "tone," the better you will look even if your weight stays temporarily the same.

The exercises that we are going to recommend should be performed while standing in as relaxed a position as you can maintain. It is important that you breathe normally while doing them. Stop between exercises and relax. When doing isometric exercises you should attempt to utilize your muscles alone, without bending the joints. Some joint motion is allowed but the less you allow, the more effective the exercise will be. Isometric exercises are also great posture improvers; as your weight comes off, your posture will begin to respond to such exercises even more noticeably.

Interestingly enough, you don't have to perform these exercises for long periods of time. In one study, after approximately eight weeks of performing an isometric exercise three times for six seconds each, three times a day, individuals had their blood pressures lowered by forty-two points—in some cases almost to normal.

Many of our patients have said to us, "Suppose I exercised and didn't diet at all. Would I still lose weight?" The answer: You probably would. And you wouldn't have to work terribly hard at exercising, either. Walking, alone, could do it. However, studies have shown that you would have to walk at least thirty minutes a day—every day. You couldn't count the walking you normally do.

And you couldn't skip a day. Our own observations have indicated that few people are prepared to make this sort of commitment... particularly when there are easier ways, as we will describe in the following pages.

But we're not saying that exercise is not important. In fact, you might find it helpful to set up regular exercise times. One of the most effective is before going to bed at night. Take five minutes and go through an exercise pattern. Gradually work up to eight or ten minutes doing simpler muscle exercises. Gradually you will work up an individualized exercise pattern. Don't look for immediate results in weight lost, but as you progress you will start to firm up those previously fatty bulges. Your skin will also begin to get more of a glow. If you find this type of exercising is too much of a drag, get into the isometric exercises we will discuss in the various chapters that follow. We have found that a combination of isometric and a few common skeletal exercises such as push-ups and straight-leg raising will help your dieting immeasurably.

SMOKING

Relax. If you are a smoker, you don't have to stop. In fact, we insist that you don't—at least not during the course of this diet. No, we aren't recommending smoking to lose weight; nor do we think the weed is particularly good for you. In fact, we'd like to see you pack in your pack, but there's a catch. Smoking, like eating, is an emotional crutch. If you throw away both your crutches at the same time, you'll fall on your face. The best advice we can give you, if you want to stop smoking, is to do that first and then go on a diet. It's admirable to want to turn over a new leaf, but that's no reason to try to turn over the whole tree. There are a number of excellent plans which you can choose among in order to stop smoking. Furthermore, the self-control you'll have learned in doing that will come to your aid in losing weight.

Other forms of oral satiation you need not give up. Chief among these is gum chewing. It would help to get a sugarless brand; if one is not available you may have to do with the sugared kind. Use half a stick at a time and don't worry too much about the sugar. The relief you get from masticating will be worth the few extra calories.

GET EIGHT HOURS OF SLEEP

You must get eight hours of sleep by the clock. If you wake up early, lie in bed until the time is up. You can read or just daydream, but you must spend the time relaxing. There are several reasons for this. First, your body can use the rest. We've taken away a number of the "quick-energy" foods and your body is going to find it necessary to get its energy from your fat deposits. It does this reluctantly; your fat deposit is to your body what your bank deposits are to you. Except, perhaps, your body is richer. During the lag period when you have cut down on these quick-energy carbohydrate calories and your body has not yet finished going through the complicated process of converting your fat to sugar, you may feel "pooped" as we have heard people on other plans put it. While this is only a temporary situation, it is still annoying. We have never known it to happen on the Nine-Day Plan; in fact, most of our patients tell us they've never had so much energy in their life as when on this regime. However, we do believe that any change in nutrition that involves a period of more than a few days should allow the body the proper energy equilibrium to accomplish the weight loss, and this is best done by giving it plenty of rest. You may feel so good on the Nine-Day Plan that you'll overdo your normal activities; this will eventually catch up with you and then you *will* feel fatigued. So make it an absolute rule, whether you think you need it or not, to get eight hours of rest per night.

Of course, there's another reason for getting this rest. When you're asleep you aren't going to be eating. You may dream about your favorite delicacies, but a diet of dreams is the most pleasant way to lose weight. In fact, sleep therapy has been in fashion among doctors in Russia as a way to reduce. Whatever success was achieved by dieting in this manner, however, seems to have diminished when the patients were fully awake, since at that time they went right back to their old eating habits. However, the basic idea isn't a bad one; you've probably done a bit of it yourself when you didn't want to eat and went to bed early. So, go to bed and get the eight hours: better eight than ate. Take a book...turn on the TV (the greatest soporific we know)...and pleasant dreams.

DEFEAT BOREDOM

What defeats most people on any diet plan is boredom. You get tired of the same routine, the same foods, the same instructions day after day after day. And no wonder. Studies done in controlling weight loss in teenagers show that a highly ritualized regime may be successful initially, but the individual will be fat again in a year or so. As physicians, we've found that the best way to help patients lose weight is to keep one step ahead of them. Therefore, we offer you, our "patients," a plan that is not only different from other diets, but even different from itself on a day-to-day basis, with as little of the routine about it as possible. If you follow this diet, you can lose anywhere from eight to twelve pounds in the time calculated....lose it easily, and without being bored. Since each day you will start a different portion of the plan, you are never standing in one place, but are always moving forward to get on with the great adventure of living thin.

2
THE DOS AND DONTS CHECKLIST FOR WHAT, HOW, WHEN, WHERE

A good portion of this material will be repeated as we go along, but we want to establish an early reference point as a guide to what will follow. You should look back at this part of the book from time to time; it will help you get back on the right track if you're doing something wrong, and will make a good attempt even better.

THE DOS: PLANNING

1. Get a medical checkup. Yes, we've heard about how the yearly physical may be a waste of time and money, but we're not talking about that extensive a workup. Your exam should include the doctor's listening to your heart and lungs both at rest and during exercise, an EKG and blood work that includes testing of thyroid and kidney function, blood sugar, cholesterol, gout and a complete blood count. That's not so bad and shouldn't put your purse into famine.

2. Are you going to attempt the plan solo, or is someone going to do it with you? Which is best? Frankly, we have found that the answer to this is based on the personalities of those involved. As a general rule we don't encourage husband and wife to diet together. While at first this might seem a logical notion, in reality the competition can become terrific, with the end result a disaster for both. Talk it over with your dieting partner, if such there be, and set some ground rules. For instance: no jealousy if one loses more weight than the other, no cop-outs for menstrual periods or pressures at the office and, above all, no using the dieting plan as a battleground to continue other arguments.

If you are going to be dieting solo, let everyone you are living with in on the plan. Ideally, they should be eager to help and encourage you; they can't do this if you keep them in the dark about what you are doing.

3. What is your schedule like? If you don't have nine consecutive days to devote to the Plan, just accommodating half the time won't lose you half the calculated weight. Many of our patients lost nothing for the first four or five days, getting the majority of their weight loss toward the end of the cycle. So if you've a wedding or other celebratory event coming up, wait until it is over to start your diet.

4. Compile a list of friends whom you are going to tell about your diet. Don't ad lib your news. Your friends can aid or diminish your enthusiasm based on their own personalities or *their* past dieting history. Nothing is more squelching than telling someone how you have high hopes and having him or her respond negatively. You don't need this sort of grief; the time to avoid it is at the beginning.

5. If possible, designate someone in the family as your "watchdog." This person's job is to remind you, as gently as possible, should the occasion arise when you are tempted to go off the plan, that you have every reason to stay on it. It is essential that he or she not become a nag, though; you'll end up eating then to spite your watchdog, a situation that is certainly tragic and that we have seen occur far too often. The gentler the prodding, the better. It shouldn't be a goad.

6. Always remember, you started this because you were frightened. Something made you take up arms against your weight. Stay frightened. Don't lapse into lethargy. Don't get cocky. Either feeling will lead to eventual tapering off of weight loss, gradual replacement of pounds. Use that edge of fright as a weapon to combat that other you, the fat you, the one that's always waiting to sabotage you. Remember, there's no thin person inside you trying to get out; just an even fatter one outside trying to get in.

7. Tell your family doctor that you are on a diet and explain to him just how it works. Show him this book; if he is interested in your health he should have a working knowledge of what plan you are using to lose weight. Knowing that you are on a diet plan, he will not prescribe for you medications containing sugar. At least we hope he won't; it's been our experience that many doctors don't care. They're interested only in the specific part of you they happen to be treating at the time. If that's how your doctor is relating to you, perhaps it's time you found another, one who will treat you as a person, not a symptom.

8. Determine how many cycles it will take to get you to the weight you want. We do not advise beginning a second cycle immediately after finishing a first one. You should wait at least a week between cycles, utilizing the Cycle Balancing Diets that may be found in that chapter.

ACTIVITIES

1. Each day you should review your diary notes of the day before. Pay special attention to what you ate and whether it filled you up or left you feeling unsatisfied. We have made provision for this, but you can utilize these "food bonuses" only if you are strictly honest with yourself. We have tried to tailor this plan to as many individual differences in capacity and desire as possible. Compare your fast days, one with the next, and see how you feel now as compared with the last.

2. These diary notes should include, for eating days, the amount you eat (even though we have clearly stated the allotted amount, you may find yourself eating more—or less—when you check it out), the time of eating (again, you may find yourself not sticking to the time we give you), the place you are eating in (what room in the house or, if you are eating out, where? A restaurant? A friend's house?) and what your state of mind is when eating. Are you angry that you're on a diet? Do you resent the fast days? Do you feel rejected by your family and friends? Are you just dieting to prove to yourself how useless it all is? Many chronic dieters do just this and use their predestined failure as an excuse to eat and get fatter. Constantly making notes and analyzing your state of mind will help you understand not only why you always failed before but how, if you really want to succeed, this time you can—by changing your previous behavior.

3. During the nine-day cycle, when you eat at home try to confine your eating to a single room in the house. It may be the kitchen, it may be the dining room. Don't forget what room you ate in last; marking it down in your diary will be an easy reference. Even if your family is eating in another room, you should stick to the one you have selected as your "home" room. The members of your family, knowing this, can help. In order not to have you eat alone and feel "different" from everyone else, they can adapt to your necessity in this respect.

4. Use the same color place mat, napkin, plate, silverware, for every meal. Sit in the same place at the table. Avoid making mealtime a "big deal." You're the only "big deal" you have to worry about. Eating should be just another of the day's activities. Talk to any of your thin friends. If they are really naturally thin and not secret dieters, they'll tell you that mealtimes, to them, are just times of the day like any other times. They don't watch the clock, counting the minutes till lunch or dinner. Many of them miss meals, they're so uninvolved with food as a thing in itself. When was the last time you missed a meal...and didn't feel a glow of pride, self-achievement? Your thin friends can miss meals without batting an eye because to them there's nothing special about eating.

We want you, too, to make food, if not "nothing" special, at least less special. By investing meals with extra frills, framing them out with ornate table decorations and so on, you elevate the mood of the hour. This will increase your appetite, which responds to such external stimuli, and you'll eat more. Think back to the ambience of many restaurants: the semidarkness (which also hides the food, allowing you to eat more since what you don't see can't hurt you), the gleaming silverware, freshly laundered tablecloths, flowers. Even if you weren't hungry when you came in, the atmosphere provokes gluttony.

Ever eat in a restaurant where the tablecloth was spotted and stained? Where the walls were peeling and the chairs were uncomfortable? Chances are you'd have eaten less. We're not telling you to run out and savage your house, but do realize that even a diamond responds to its setting and increases its value in the eye of the beholder. The same is true for food. Look at any of the ads in the gourmet magazines. The decor makes your mouth water. Take the same foods, space them out individually by pasting their pictures on ordinary paper with a white background, and you'll see the difference. So, even though it may sound peculiar, don't invest your eating precincts with any more appetizing arrays than the food itself.

5. Feel free to go on vacation. Many people consider vacations in the nature of extended weekends and resign themselves to going off whatever diet they may be on at the time and to come home looking, as one of our patients put it, "like something the cat dragged in if the cat was a tiger." But, by the very nature of the vacation, you will not be home, not at the mercy of the refrigerator, not (in many instances) able to eat at will but only when the dining room is open. Even if you are cooking for yourself and the family, chances are that you will be spending a lot of time exploring your new surroundings and thinking less about food. You are also likely to be exercising more than at home—either on the tennis court, in the swimming pool, horseback riding, hiking, or such. One thing you may do is drink more alcohol than you would at home. This you must be careful of. Otherwise, the Nine-Day Wonder Diet is just as Wonderful away from home, possibly even more so. Don't, therefore, be afraid to take a vacation. You've got it coming; you deserve it. You don't deserve to be fat, however, so wherever you go, take us along and when you get home you'll be astonished at all the weight you didn't gain. In fact you'll come home lighter, not heavier. Won't that be great?

CONTROL OF EATING BEHAVIOR

1. Eat more slowly. You probably have never considered it, but chances are you're a fast eater. Most fat people are. You can easily tell if speed's your problem by timing yourself. Put a stopwatch on the table. You may be shocked to find out how quickly you polish off your plate. The faster you eat, the more you'll eat because you aren't satisfying the hunger of your mouth. All you are doing is filling your stomach. The fact is, your stomach can be full and you can still be left with mouth hunger. We all do it. How many times have you had a Chinese meal and been hungry an hour or so afterward though you were full at the time you ate? And you'll say, "Boy, that stuff was light, it went right through me." Yet you haven't had a bowel movement and you don't see noodles dropping out of your pores. Where did the food go? It's still there, still in your stomach, where it will remain for from three to four hours. Then why are you hungry? Because it slid right down; you ate it so fast that you never gave your mouth a chance to get into the act.

All of us, fat and thin, are orally fixated to some extent. Food is especially important in this respect because your mouth was built to chew and taste. All the taste buds in your body, the instruments of which gourmets sing, are crowded into a small portion of your tongue. And your tongue is in your mouth. So, eating fast, you aren't really giving yourself a chance to enjoy the flavor of the food. Instead, you are eating with your eyes and your stomach, using your mouth as a convenient passageway between the two. This leaves your mouth feeling hungry and yourself unsatisfied, apt to "nibble," "snack," "cheat," and all the other words you use when you are sneakily trying to undo the damage you caused to yourself at mealtimes. The best way to undo this damage is to learn to eat slowly. There are a few techniques that will apply here:

A. Chew your food until it is a liquid in your mouth. This does a number of things. First, it prevents you from gobbling huge clumps of food directly into your stomach, acquiring heartburn in the process since your stomach is not equipped to handle them. Proper chewing process mixes your food with saliva, which begins the digestion process in your mouth. Despite what you may think, the saliva isn't there just to "wash down" your food, though it helps there too. We've actually seen people gobbling so fast that they weren't able to manufacture a quantity of saliva rapidly enough to grease their palates; such individuals would use quantities of soda or beer to help get the food into their stomachs. Ever see a pizza- or spaghetti-eating contest on TV? It's quite a spectacle. The fattest contestant usually wins: he's the fastest eater.

If you eat slowly, chewing your food until it is a liquid and allowing the proper flow of saliva, your food begins to be digested by your body. The digestive process starts in the mouth, so make sure you chew. If, initially, you have to go so far as to count the bites, do that. Concentrate on eating. Our entire plan, unlike other diets, is aimed at getting you to do exactly this: concentrate on *eating,* not on *not eating.*

B. Count each mouthful. In addition to counting how much chewing you do, know how many times that fork is going up. We don't really care what the total is; we simply want you to realize what is happening, that the eating experience is occurring.

C. Put your eating utensils down on the plate after every mouthful. Few people do this and yet it is a good idea. First, it helps you concentrate on what you've already got in your mouth, rather than what is to come. It also slows you down because, once you are ready for the next mouthful, you have to pick up your utensils again and realize that you are indulging in the eating experience. This constant reminder to yourself may sound like a fairly simplistic idea, but think back. How many times have you eaten something and not even remember doing so? This happens because the eating process, once started, becomes mechanical for most people. The rhythm becomes hypnotic, deceitful. We rock ourselves with it to fantasyland, where our constant cry is, "But I don't eat that much." Compared to whom? Compared to *you,* obviously you do. The evidence is right before your eyes. So is the food, if you have the eyes to see it. . .and the honesty to chalk it up. . .and the guidance to slow it down.

D. When you eat, sit down. Never eat standing up. Whenever you've eaten standing up in the past, you've been in a hurry. You had to pick someone up at the airport, get the kids to school, meet a date, pick up your car, run to the PTA, get to a movie. Eating, then, became a job to get over. You'll eat more standing at a buffet, walking around, talking to people, mindlessly reaching out for those provocative nibbles, than you will, seated, for a three- or four-course meal. If you "haven't the time" to sit down to eat, you "haven't the time" to eat. Period. Every meal plan in this book is meant to be eaten sitting down. *Whatever you eat, eat it sitting down.* There seems to be a mistaken notion among some individuals that by standing or walking about while eating, they tend to burn off more of the calories going in. This is just another "fat" excuse. No way will it happen. By sitting down you make every snack into a meal and you know very well that meals count. Snacks don't count, right? It's only a snack, after all, you tell yourself. How much can it matter? But a meal? You've never been able to convince yourself that *that* doesn't matter. By sitting down, turning everything you eat into a formal meal, you will be able to convince yourself, rather rapidly, that everything you put into your mouth matters.

E. Interrupt the eating experience. There are several ways to accomplish this. You might eat one portion of the meal, such as the meat, then pause, get up from the table, look out the window, do something constructive such as kick the dog, then go back to the next portion, perhaps the vegetables. Eating this way, in spurts, goes against everything we've been told since childhood. "Sit down and finish your meal," our mothers used to reprimand us. "Don't get up from the table again until you're done." Yet we have found that interrupting the meal is a necessity for the fat person. It allows you to take a breath, lets your mouth catch up with your stomach, wakens you from "eating hypnotism." Even the act of going back for seconds—physically getting up and going over to the stove to take them from the pot—is psychologically filling. Just that much interruption of the eating propulsion may allow you to realize that you aren't really still hungry. After all, how many times have you gotten a phone call during a meal, come back to the table after a few moments speaking to the caller and found that you'd "lost your appetite"? What you had done, accidentally, was to shake yourself out of the eating stupor that prods all of us to finish whatever we put on our plates. You can't always arrange a phone call at the opportune time, but you can build into each meal enough of a staccato quality to keep you always aware of how much you are eating as opposed to how hungry you think you really are.

F. Take small portions. Start off on our menus with less than we advise wherever you can. That way you accomplish two things. First, you leave yourself something to fall back on if you're still really hungry. Second, by going for more you interrupt your eating hypnosis and just maybe will find that you don't want it after all. Don't deny yourself if you do want more; our diet has been carefully calculated to accomplish the proper weight loss for you, but there is, all the same, a great deal of variation from person to person, so that what would quite fill A might leave B unsatisfied. We don't want that to happen and have taken great pains to guard against it. Naturally, once you put "seconds" on your plate, you return to the table. You always have a round-trip ticket. Never stand at the stove eating out of the pot. You'll eat the whole thing.

G. Learn when you're hungry and when you're full. Sound simple? When was the last time you asked yourself? One of the problems we ran into when testing the Nine-Day Plan was that people thought they *had* to eat all the food we listed. As one patient put it, "I guess I wasn't really hungry, but I can always eat. I just never fill up." Let us, therefore, first caution you that on this plan you *do not have to* eat everything that is listed for the various days. At the same time, if you are hungry, the food is there for you. When are you hungry and when are you full? The way to start learning the answer to this is by asking yourself, every time you sit down to eat, "Am I hungry, really hungry? Would I eat something I don't really care for?" If the answer—in all honesty—is yes, chances are that you are hungry. If, at the same time, your stomach is uncomfortable (not "growling"; despite what many people think, that isn't a sign of hunger) and your mouth feels empty, such physical signs are definite backups to the hunger process. However, if you eat just because the food is available, or because it happens to be that time of day, or because you feel you are socially obligated to do so, you will never lose weight no matter how many diets you go on. Most of your fat is in your head. Unless you lose it there, no matter how often you lose it elsewhere it will always return.

THE DON'TS: PLANNING

1. Don't choose an unrealistic goal. Far too often people not only want to lose below what they should, but they frustrate themselves trying to get there and make themselves sick in the process. Your ideal weight is very much determined by your own characteristics as an individual. Just because a friend of yours weighs 110 pounds, that doesn't mean *you* have to. Your weight-loss factor should be calculated according to your present weight, height and age, your caloric and nutritional needs, your level of physical activity, your overall physical condition, the kinds of food you prefer and have eaten in the past and your ethnic background. Each of these factors will be a vital check on how low you can go, and if there's any question in your mind you should discuss the matter with your family physician.

2. Don't let someone talk you into losing weight. Your weight-loss program must be your own idea. If you are shamed into it by the nagging of your spouse, or get involved just so that your friends and family will get off your back, you'll have the same resistance to it that you would to forced feeding. No one can make up your mind as to what you ought to do with your own body. You may be perfectly contented being fat; there's no law against it, and certainly, to attempt to get thin just to oblige other people not only won't work, but out of sheer frustration you'll end up eating more and will likely get even fatter. Adolescents are especially prone to "secondhand" dieting: losing weight because they are forced into it by their parents. And while the concert halls are full of great musicians who were forced by their parents to practice when they were children, we've never known an individual who got thin strictly from parental or any other outside pressure... and stayed that way. So examine the reasons why you want to lose weight. What are your motivations? Are they sound? If you are doing it to please someone else, or to keep your job, or because the weather is changing, chances are that you will *lose* weight—certainly on the Nine-Day Wonder Diet—but your chances of *keeping it off* will be far better if you are doing it basically for yourself, because you know that what you want is a better life being thin.

3. Don't make yourself out to be perfect. Nobody is. But because you may feel you've had so many years being imperfect—that is, fat—you may feel that you should now be absolutely "good" about losing. The first time you go off the plan—and people do go off the plan; we realize it and expect it—you will feel ashamed, embarrassed, confirmed as being the unworthy person you always knew you were. You aren't unworthy. You are expecting too much from yourself. You wouldn't expect it from anyone else. What would you say to a friend in your situation? "Don't be foolish. You know this diet you are on works; you've already lost weight on it. Just forget about this setback and go back on it." And that's what you must tell yourself. This doesn't mean you should be approaching the Nine-Day Plan expecting failure. That's a sure way to disaster, as we have discussed. But expecting yourself to be perfect is another way to court failure.

4. Don't engage in other activities while eating. When you eat, eat. Become involved with your food to the exclusion of all else. Don't watch TV, argue with the family (the hotter the argument, the faster you'll eat), read or talk on the phone. If eating is important to you, and it must be because here you are, then it is an activity worth concentrating on. Otherwise you begin to dilute the experience and you won't remember what you ate, how you ate or, indeed, if you ate at all. Compare this with making a purchase in a department store. All the while you are choosing your merchandise there is music playing in the background. You leave the store after half an hour or an hour—can you recall one tune that was played? It's unlikely that you can. The music was playing all the time and your ear caught it, but you only heard it subliminally, unconsciously, as a background. If you treat your food that way, using it as a background to more intense activities, you'll wonder why your foreground is getting bigger.

5. Don't get carried away by the amount of weight you lose. We have had people on the Nine-Day Plan who have lost fourteen, eighteen and twenty-two pounds within the allotted time. You may be one of them. But don't then start believing you've found a magic cure, that you can put on weight again and lose it at will. Eventually, you will find that your weight loss will begin to slow down and, if you aren't careful, the plan will not work nearly as well—for you specifically, that is, because you've abused it. We recommend several cycles of the diet, depending on how much weight you have to lose, but it is that first cycle that usually loses the most weight for you. If you maintain your weight loss on the Cycle Balancing Diets, then go back on the Nine-Day Plan; you will continue to lose. But if you go right back to your old eating habits between cycles, you will find a great disillusion awaiting you when you go back to the plan. Maybe not the second or third time, but sooner or later your body will balk.

6. Don't call yourself names. You aren't a fat slob, you don't eat garbage and you aren't a cheater. Whether or not other people think so, you certainly don't have to agree with them. We don't, and we can't let you, because calling yourself all these essentially bad things means that you are a hopeless case, not worth saving. And we and you know that isn't true. If it were, you wouldn't be reading this book, trying to do a job that is one of the toughest in the world. In our office we tell our patients never to call us "fat doctors." First of all, neither of us is fat... anymore. We were at one time, but we lost our weight according to our own plan. That was many years ago—thirteen for one of us, seven for the other—and we've never gained the weight back, nor do we intend to. But we have a more pertinent reason for telling our patients that we aren't "fat doctors." We don't treat fat. We treat people. We've never had a pound of fat come walking solus through our office door. There's always been a person attached to it. So we're people doctors—and that's one of the things that makes our plan different from all others. All the other diets treat fat. But fat can't hear, read or understand. Only people can. And only people can change one life-style for another—if they really want to.

7. Don't expect rewards for what you're not doing. It's basic human nature to want to get paid for a job well done. But the payment for this particular job is down the road apiece, not immediately 'round the corner. You know that, yet all the same you can't help thinking, "Shouldn't I have *some* reward for all those things I'm not eating?" Your reward, of course, comes in pounds and inches lost, but often that isn't enough. Not long ago Mary Jane L. was in our office. She'd been on the Nine-Day Plan for almost a week and had lost seven pounds, more than she'd done in a comparable time span on any other diet she'd tried—and Mary Jane had tried them all. Nonetheless, she was disappointed. "Is that all?" she huffed. "It should have been more." When we pointed out to her that she still had three important days to go and besides, we asked her, by whose rules should it be more, her answer was: "I've been so good this week." We thereupon told her this story.

When we were in general practice we had a young lady come in who'd missed three menstrual periods. After being examined and told she was pregnant, her response was similar: "How could I be pregnant? I've been so good this week."

Mary Jane got the message.

ACTIVITIES

1. Remember, don't overweigh yourself. The temptation is always there, but you'll drive yourself crazy; nothing will happen fast enough and you'll just get discouraged. The best thing is to stay away from the scale entirely during at least the first three or four days. Remember, most of your weight will probably be lost later in the diet rather than early on or in the middle.

2. Don't under- or overdo your exercising. We have indicated in the course of the Plan what type of exercising to do and for how long. However, as in the case of amounts of food, you may want more exercise than we provide. That's fine. But, on the other hand, if you go overboard you can end up in trouble, the least of which will amount to sore muscles and joints. Then you'll blame us. Exercising, other than what we recommend—and we recommend the minimal so that everyone will be able to join in—should be a personal program planned according to your specific needs, tastes and abilities. If you put yourself through too rigorous a program you will only get discouraged and this may undermine your entire diet plan. Keep in mind that there are individual exercises as well as group exercises and though you, as an overweight person, may not be comfortable in such group exercises as softball or tennis or bowling, you can still stick to such individual exercise activities as jogging, gardening, swimming, calisthenics and, of course, walking. Got a dog? That's the best way to walk. Especially if you've a big dog. You'll be pulling back on the leash in addition to trying to keep up with him or having him keep up with you. Few professional dog walkers are fat.

3. Don't be thrown by periods of crisis. Illness or death in the family usually gets the overweight person even fatter. This is understandable—and reversible if you only make the effort to get off the merry-go-round of hospital and family visits once the crisis is over. There are some individuals who can't eat at all when they are upset. They are in the minority. Most of us, faced with a crisis, run to food as a universal pacifier. If you allow the crisis life-style to continue once the crisis is over, then you should blame yourself. But, remember, you can always change it today instead of tomorrow.

4. Don't be embarrassed to come back to us. We'll always be here, in these pages, waiting for you. We know what's happened before: you've taken off weight, determined to finish the job; then something happened and there you are, fat again, discouraged again, still determined to lose, but you think you're a failure. Our Plan, which worked so well for you before—will it work again? Perhaps you should try something else, something that promises you more even if you don't know if it can deliver.

Our advice is to come back to a plan that you know works. If it's your second attempt, or even your third, perhaps you won't have the quick results of your first, but results will still come. It may take you more cycles to lose, but at least you'll be losing in a safe, logical, healthy manner—and chances are that whatever weight you've gained, you're not as fat as you were when you started.

But even if you are, don't be embarrassed to come back to us. Anyone can show off a success. The tough part isn't fiddling around, it's facing the music. Re-losing the weight you've gained shouldn't be an occasion for embarrassment but rather one for reaffirmation, a new resolve to be thin. Remember, you're not a failure unless you quit entirely. There are no other failures on our Plan. As long as you are doing something about your problem you can't possibly be a failure. Both of us have been discouraged over our weight; we've both been fat. We know how you feel, and we know how easy it is to quit. It's as easy as getting fat.

3
THE NINE-DAY WONDER DIET GIVES YOU QUICK WEIGHT LOSS

Quick weight loss is what you are after. You'll also lose inches where you want to see them go; those unsightly bumps and bulges will begin to flatten out and firm up as you follow this plan. An executive of a large corporation told us, after losing fifteen pounds in nine days, that if he had his way he would make this plan mandatory in his factory. We've had airline hostesses on the Nine-Day Plan. Many of them had gotten fat after the airlines had lifted weight restrictions. They needed to get thin again in a hurry. You may feel the same urgency, and you, too, can lose your weight easily and rapidly.

THE VALUE OF QUICK WEIGHT LOSS

It isn't true (as many people, hoping to comfort themselves, think) that the faster you lose weight, the faster you'll put it back on. We've had patients on this diet who have stayed thin for years. The fact is, the faster you lose your weight, especially if you've got only fifteen to twenty pounds to lose, the better you'll feel, the higher your morale will be and the more efficiently you'll be able to handle your weight-loss situation. We want you to get on with the job, get it over with and get ahead with the business of living—a business that has lost a lot of its zip since you got to be overweight.

31

If you've more than twenty pounds to lose, chances are you're already a three- or four-time "loser" and pretty discouraged with all the previous diets you've tried. The Nine-Day Plan has been calculated for you as well as for the individual who has much less to lose. By demonstrating to you that you *can* lose weight—and rapidly—we will convince you that you are far from the hopeless case you might well consider yourself. After a few cycles of the Nine-Day-Plan you will be able to combine it with sustained periods on our Food Intake Plan (FIP, described in our previous book *You Can Be Fat Free Forever,* available at your local bookstore or from St. Martin's Press in New York City). You will be as astonished as the high school principal who went on our Plan and told us that in twenty years of involvement in education, this was the most important thing *he'd* been taught. And it is astonishing. Wait until you total up the pounds you've lost and the amount of time saved. Nothing succeeds like success and if you are serious about losing weight, success with this Plan is just around the corner. All you need do is follow the simple, clear instructions and you'll turn that corner.

WHY WE START ON THE WEEKEND

Traditionally, the weekend is when most dieters do their cheating, go off their plan, are "bad" so they'll have something to reproach themselves with on Monday morning. We're going to give you something else to talk about Monday—a diet you not only can stick to over the weekend, but one that won't cramp your weekend style of living. It's fun for us, when we present new patients with this plan, to watch the look on their faces and hear them say something like, "Start this on Saturday? Well, I guess that will pretty well cool my calendar." Nine days later, when they come in to be weighed, they bring rave notices. "You know," a typical remark will be, "this is the first time I could take a diet and do just about everything I normally do on a weekend and not feel hemmed in." And in a moment or two the patient will add: "And I lost weight, too."

The purpose of starting and ending this Plan on a weekend—the time involved includes two weekends and the five days between—is simple but unique. There is the effect of surprise. You've always considered dieting a form of punishment. It needn't be. We want to get that idea out of your head; we want you to consider this Plan a totally different experience from anything you've had before. Most people use the weekend as a time of rest and relaxation. Isn't that the best time to consider what you are going to do about your weight? Haven't you more time then to seek out your motivations for losing weight and to put the principles of weight loss into practice than during the hectic days of the week, when you have more than enough pressures and will likely add going on a diet to them; just one more pressure you can be relieved of when the weekend comes?

We have calculated the two weekends and five weekdays so as to utilize your life-style to best advantage—to make your normal routines work for, rather than against, your new diet plan. In this manner we hope to make your diet mesh with all your other activities. You should have more energy, not less, under this regime and, provided you follow all instructions exactly, you should lose between eight to twelve pounds *on your first cycle!*

THE CYCLICAL NATURE OF THE PLAN

Eight to twelve pounds may be all you have to lose, so that one cycle on the Nine-Day Plan will restore you to normal and will probably be all you need to start living thin for the rest of your life. However, we must tell you that to keep yourself that way you will have to change some of the eating habits that got you fat in the first place. We will discuss methods by which this may be accomplished as we go into the individual days. Let us say you've more than twelve pounds to lose but less than twenty. One cycle may still do for you; we have patients who have lost over eighteen pounds during their first cycle on the Nine-Day Plan. But let's say you are not one of them. You have several choices. You can use the Nine-Day Plan as a quick start toward your ideal weight and go from there on to any other diet plan of your choice. You can let a few weeks go by and get on a second cycle of the Nine-Day Plan. During the time between your first and second cycles, you should be on our Cycle Balancing Diet, which you will find in Chapter 13, along with modifications of this basic Plan. And, again, if you are truly obese, with anywhere from fifty to a hundred pounds to lose, we recommend combining the Nine-Day Plan with our Food Intake Plan to lose weight rapidly over a much longer time period.

WHY WE DEVISED THE NINE-DAY PLAN

In our office we treat only the obese—that is, patients who weigh at least twenty pounds more than their normal weight. We have been treating such individuals for years with great success, and turning away all those who came to us for help who were not that heavy. Some time ago a woman came into the office and asked us if we didn't recognize her voice. It seems she'd called the office repeatedly to seek our help for her weight problem but she wasn't heavy enough to be allowed to come. "When I first called," she told us, "I was about eight pounds over my normal weight. When I called again I was thirteen pounds past what I should have weighed. Now look at me." Her weight that evening showed her twenty-five pounds over normal. "You might say," she added reproachfully, "that I finally ate my way into your office. You could have saved me a lot of grief, time and money if you'd seen me sooner."

This incident started us thinking. Checking with our receptionist, we found that she was turning away dozens of people a day because, according to our rules, they were not heavy enough to justify our seeing them. But was this attitude of ours correct? Should these people literally have to eat themselves into our attention? Wouldn't it be better to short-circuit the process, catch them before they got really obese? We thought this notion worthy of pursuit and began doing research on the subject. Then using our patients, all of whom were enthusiastic about the idea, we proceeded to try out a new diet plan. We found that with the very obese the Nine-Day Plan alone, while it produced a rapid weight loss, was not sustaining enough for the total poundage these individuals had to lose. It was of value, however, in combination with the plan they were already on—our Food Intake Plan—when used at judicious intervals. However, with people who had only from five to twenty or even thirty pounds to lose, the Nine-Day Plan not only took off large amounts of weight quickly and painlessly, but when we combined it with certain principles of our Food Intake Plan based on behavior modification, these patients did not regain their weight.

So it is no longer necessary for you to have to eat your way into our office. Our office is right here, in these pages. Just open the cover and come on in. You'll come out with results you may have long hoped for but never been able to realize—at least that's what our happy patients have said to us.

Why You Can Lose Weight This Way
Even If You're A Three- or Four-Time Loser

We've had plenty of "dietary deficiencies" on this Plan. That's what one of our patients called himself. "The diets I've been on aren't deficient," he told us, "I am." Our answer was that we didn't believe him; that anyone who recognized he had a weight problem and was attempting to remedy that problem, far from being "deficient," was behaving most rationally. "But I just can't seem to stick to them," he confessed. "It's the same thing over and over. Each day is monotonous and eventually I go on a binge and eat my way right up the wall." This is only normal. Variation is a way of life. You wouldn't care to go to the same picture show over and over, and most divorces come about because of sheer monotony. If this is enough to separate a person from his or her spouse, certainly it's enough to cause you to part company with a boring diet. Unfortunately, due to their very nature, most diets are just that—boring. We've rectified this situation by varying your daily activity with food; by not taking away from you all the things you may love; and, where we have had to prohibit certain items, by attempting to replace them with tasty, if not caloric, equals. Most important, you won't be doing the same thing day after day. On the nine days on this Plan you will be faced with changes of pace as well as changes of palate. Our aim is to keep you on your toes—while causing you to shed enough weight so as to stay there.

WHY IT IS SAFE AND HEALTHY
TO LOSE WEIGHT THIS WAY

If you were to go on a diet of oxtail soup for a year, you probably would have some difficulty in adjusting and end up in a nutritive disaster. But if you were to go on such a diet for only a day, while you might not lose much weight, you'd scarcely be doing yourself any harm. Well, we don't offer you oxtail soup on the Nine-Day

Plan, but there are some things we tell you to do that, if carried to extremes, could get you into trouble. *Fasting,* for instance. If you did this for months at a clip without medical supervision, it could be dangerous. For the two separated days we ask you to do it on the Nine-Day Plan, however, it will help you lose a lot of weight and do you no harm at all.

If you ate only the *protein foods* we advise without any supplements and for an extended period, your body would be deprived of essential nutrients. But we don't ask you to do that; furthermore, during the course of this Plan, we tell you to take certain supplemental backups. These are more to help you with your weight loss than to make up for anything you might be lacking in the diet. The two days of protein eating not only won't hurt you, not only will help you lose weight, but will furnish your body with a goodly supply of the amino acids it needs to stay healthy and keep your energy up.

HIDDEN CALORIES

In general, the foods in this diet have not only been carefully chosen for variety and nutritive value, but their methods of preparation have been delineated so that you can avoid "hidden" calories. What are hidden calories? The difference between a large apple and small one can be as much as seventy calories, though as far as your body is concerned the vitamin and mineral content is the same. This is because your body gets rid of the extra vitamins and minerals it cannot use, but it stores the extra calories in the form of fat.

Let's take another example. A meal consisting of a pork chop, broccoli, mashed potatoes, a frozen dessert, peaches and coffee can be prepared so that it contains 850 calories, or so that it contains 1,500 calories. Appearance and protein content may be exactly the same, but sauces and mode of preparation can kill your diet. How? Well, a pork chop that is baked rather than fried saves 260 calories; a yogurt rather than a sour cream sauce on the broccoli saves 140 calories; only one tablespoon of butter in the potato, rather than two, knocks off another 100 calories. If the dessert is ice milk rather than ice cream, with sugar-free canned peaches instead of peaches with syrup, there's another 80 calories you won't be ingesting. These are hidden calories: the price of unthinking food preparation. What have you sacrificed by not utilizing these hidden calories? Very little, really. You've indulged your taste buds; you can't say you are being forced to eat "special" foods or can't go out to eat; what you've had is nutritious and wholesome and satisfying—and you've lost weight without going hungry. The way your food is prepared will, of itself, lose you anywhere from two to three pounds during the nine-day period if you do nothing else the Plan calls for. Of course, during this time we're going to be constantly at your elbow, "spoon-feeding" you, if you will, according to the diets in this book. But, *when you finish your cycle, don't misplace the lessons we hope you will have learned about food.* That is one of the ways you'll stay thin.

There are other ways to diminish hidden calories. Trim most of the fat from your meats and use meat that itself is not fatty. Always broil or bake rather than fry. Anytime you are taking milk in quantity—as in a glassful, for instance—use skim rather than whole milk. Salad dressings have to be carefully watched; use a minimum.

This does not mean that your meals will be dull or bland or monotonous. One way to keep them from being so is to use condiments. All the spices are at your disposal, as well as lemon juice, which is good on meats as well as fish and vegetables and which, for some reason, is rarely so used.

SALT

Unfortunately, this is one condiment that you must be wary of. Salt is sodium chloride and your body tries to hold as much sodium as it can. In doing this, it must also hold a lot of water. So if you are a heavy salt taker you must learn to stop. This goes for onion, garlic and celery salt as well: such mixtures contain real salt. However, onion or garlic powder, as well as onion or garlic cloves, are fine. "I salt everything," one patient confided to us, "even Lipton's Noodle Soup." All one can do is wince in the face of such a confession.

Most people have rather a mystical feeling about salt. They attribute powers to it that it does not have; the taking of salt tablets in the summer, for instance, when one perspires heavily, is a common but unnecessary activity. You have to remember that it is only the water from your body that evaporates; the salt stays behind. As we have already indicated, your body is very possessive about salt; you needn't cater to a prejudice that is quite capably imposed as it is! If you do, you will find yourself heavier. Not fatter, for there are no calories in salt, but weighing more because of the water your body is retaining. Learn to use pepper instead of salt. It is not nearly so overpowering to the taste buds and adds immeasurably to the flavor of your food. Monosodium glutamate, much favored in Chinese and Japanese cooking, is similarly to be avoided for, as its name implies, it contains the same element—sodium—as does salt.

WHAT ABOUT ALCOHOL?

What *about* it? Well, there are quite a few calories about it: 168 of them. This is the amount you will take in from two ounces of a hundred-proof drink. A typical alcoholic drink can provide you with anywhere from just under a hundred to over three hundred calories. Again, many people like to feel, wistfully perhaps, that drinking is not eating. One patient who had had her jaws wired came to us in some distress demanding to know why she was gaining weight when obviously she wasn't eating. She was, however, drinking. Not only alcohol but quantities of fruit juices, soda and even a noodle pudding which she had put into a Waring blender, liquefied and sipped through a straw. You may laugh at this and think, "How silly." But to this lady, her perplexity was real enough. Remember, if what you are drinking contains calories—in other words, if it's anything but water—these must be taken into account on any diet plan.

The following table will give you some idea of the number of calories you can take in from some of the more common alcoholic beverages:

12 oz. of beer ....**150** calories
3−4 oz. of wine ....**85** calories
3−4 oz. of sweet wine ....**160** calories
1½ oz. of vodka ....**90** calories

```
1½ oz. of gin . . . . . . . . . . . . . . . . . . . . . . . . 106 calories
1½ oz. of whiskey  . . . . . . . . . . . . . . . . . . . 129 calories
1½ oz. of rum . . . . . . . . . . . . . . . . . . . . . . . 130 calories
1 daiquiri . . . . . . . . . . . . . . . . . . . . . . . . . . . 120 calories
1 eggnog  . . . . . . . . . . . . . . . . . . . . . . . . . . 335 calories
1 manhattan . . . . . . . . . . . . . . . . . . . . . . . 164 calories
1 mint julep . . . . . . . . . . . . . . . . . . . . . . . . 183 calories
1 old-fashioned . . . . . . . . . . . . . . . . . . . . . 179 calories
1 planter's punch . . . . . . . . . . . . . . . . . . . . 175 calories
1 Tom Collins . . . . . . . . . . . . . . . . . . . . . . . 180 calories
```

Most people tend to have more than one drink. If you are at a party you may have considerably more than that, with each containing much more than the minimum quantity described in the table. You can readily understand, then, how alcohol can add greatly to your already expanded waistline. How do you handle this? Well, on the Nine-Day Plan we are going to permit you alcohol on certain days. You certainly don't *have* to drink it if you don't want to, but for many people, just knowing it is available if they want it is enough. We do have to limit your consumption, however, to one drink only, and in the specified amount.

But what do you do if you are at a party? The best thing is to fake it. Have your one drink if you so desire, then switch to plain club soda on ice with a dash of lemon and a twist. No one is going to ask to taste it. In fact, no one will bother you as long as you don't make an issue of it. You will be treated as part of the group. Just don't set it down or some fatuous good samaritan will bring you a real drink and probably stand around to make sure that you drink it.

Remember, your overindulgence in alcohol won't necessarily add to the life of the party, but it may well contribute to the death of your diet. Weddings are particularly insidious in this regard. You may feel that unless you repeatedly toast the bride and groom with a drink, their marriage will end up on the rocks. They can probably destroy each other with or without your good wishes, and chances are you'll still be carrying the weight you gained at their wedding as you raise your glass at their divorce party.

USING FOOD ITSELF TO CONTROL YOUR WEIGHT

You will find that you will have plenty to eat on the Nine-Day Plan. At the same time, you will probably find there are a number of foods that have been omitted. Most of these have been found to be problem foods—foods that in themselves act as eating cues, or appetizers, if you will. Studies have shown that some of the greatest instigators in this regard are coffee ice cream, freshly baked chocolate chip cookies, brownies, potato chips, peanut butter, soda pop and salted peanuts. These items not only tend to instigate an eating pattern, but once you start on them it is almost impossible to stop. Potato chips and dip are a classic source of runaway joy. In fact, a popular commercial idealizing potato chips makes a point of stating, "You can't eat just one." You may call these "junk foods," but only after you've consumed the lot. The sad fact is, you just can't start on them. Once you do, they start on you and you're right back in trouble. Recognize them for what they are—disaster zones—and stay clear of them.

There is another way to think about foods, and that is in terms of the amount of purchase value you get from them. For instance, you can drink eight ounces of Coca-Cola and get as many calories as from nine ounces of skim milk, five ounce of whole milk, two ounces of Half and Half or two ounces of a chocolate milkshake. Considering only fluid quantity it would be better to drink the Coke, since it will fill you up more from the standpoint of sheer volume. Incidentally, it's a good idea to count the swallows when you drink and, of course, to drink slowly.

But let's get back to this idea of purchase value. When you drink the Coke, what do you get for your money? Actually, zero nutrition plus an ever-increasing thirst that will make you drink even more of it. Match this against the proteins, vitamins, minerals and fat content contained in the milk drinks. No comparison.

There is a way, though, by which you can get the volume of fluid you need to keep you from being constantly hungry while you are learning to control your eating pattern, and at the same time maintain proper nutrition. The miracle drink that will do this for you?

40

WATER IS A MUST

On the Nine-Day Plan you are going to drink eight glasses of water a day. It really isn't difficult once you get used to the idea. We prefer that you drink cold water, though if you want it lukewarm or even hot we won't argue with you. The only substitute for water is seltzer or club soda; not coffee or tea, and certainly not milk.

Most overweight people drink very little water. If you are already a water drinker, good for you—you are already one step ahead of almost everyone else. Keep drinking. Naturally, we don't want you drinking all this water at once. Not long ago we got a call from a patient who complained that she was "throwing up water." Upon inquiry it came out that she was drinking all her eight glasses in the morning, one after the other. Why did she do this? Her answer was simple: "I wanted to get it over with." Unfortunately, this is the way too many people feel about their diet. They only want to get it over with. If this is your attitude, the best advice we can give you is not to start at all. That way you'll get it over with in the fastest way possible.

Water has zero calories. It may make you temporarily heavier, but it won't make you any fatter. So drink. If necessary drink half a glass of water, then come back in ten minutes and drink the rest. Unlike camels, we humans do not store water: what goes in, comes out. (If we could persuade our bodies to treat our excess calories in the same fashion, none of us would get fat.) Even when we claim that we drink little or no water, we are taking in a certain amount through our solid food. Green vegetables are almost 98 percent water; meat is up to 70 percent water. Additional water is given off by the oxidation (burning) of food within us—when it is burned by the body for energy, fat yields over 100 grams of water for every 100 grams of fat that is burned.

But for the person on a diet who wants to stay healthy, this is not enough. Water is constantly being lost by the body. Much of it is lost by the skin through evaporation; a certain amount is lost through breathing; and, of course, the kidneys are constantly filtering water from the bloodstream.

This water loss takes place whether you are dieting or not; the effect of dieting, however, may be to cut down on many of the solid

41

foods that have been providing water intake. If you don't drink water under these circumstances you can get into trouble. A loss of only 10 percent of body water is a serious matter; a loss of 20 percent can be disastrous.

Drinking water, like dieting itself, takes time. We want you to spread your eight glasses out over the day. Think of them as medicine, the most potent diet enforcer. There are very practical reasons for wanting you to drink water. On the Nine-Day Plan you are going to be faced with a rapid Calorie Burn-Out Time—a concept we will be discussing in just a moment. The rapid burning up of your fat leaves certain residues in your bloodstream that we want you to flush out with water. In addition, the fluid volume of the water itself will help fill you up, keep you from being as hungry. The water also combines with many of the foods we will be providing you with that are fibrous; these foods swell in your stomach and help keep you from being hungry, but only if the proper amount of water is taken in. Water helps keep your mouth from getting dry and a bad taste from forming due to your rapid Calorie Burn-Out (CBO); helps keep the stool soft, so you won't become constipated; and cold water helps slow down the motions of your stomach that contribute to the feeling of hunger.

Interestingly enough, it isn't because they don't like the taste or never get thirsty that most people don't drink water. We have all become victims of a tremendous advertising campaign that has effectively substituted soda for water in our thinking. We've been brainwashed with pop art. And why not? After all, water is free but someone stands to make a buck if we drink soda. It may surprise you to learn that, even so, the human body has withstood the onslaught and remains approximately 70 percent water—not diet soda, regular soda or lemonade. So the sooner you get off the soda kick and back onto water, the better off you will be, the quicker and more efficiently you will lose weight. Remember, also, that even diet sodas, lacking as they may be in calories, do contain a lot of salt, a great number of compounds of sodium. And we have already discussed what that will do to you.

"The reason I don't drink water," one schoolteacher recently told us, "is not because I don't like it but because it continually

makes me have to go to the bathroom. And I can't leave my class."
We hear this all the time, and not only from schoolteachers but from
secretaries, housewives, nurses... women in all walks of life. Not so
much from men. Well, ladies, has water become a sexist liquid? In a
way, yes. Especially in women who have borne children.

To begin with, the urinary bladders of most women are smaller
then men's and thus store less water. Even so, this would not
account for the fact that when you, as a woman, take a sip of water,
you immediately feel that you have to go to the bathroom. And,
you know, very little comes out. In many women who have given
birth, the urinary bladder takes a certain amount of trauma—plain
old pounding from the baby's head coming through below. Above
the bladder are the front bones of your pelvis, the pubes. Caught
between the baby's head below and the pubes above, the bladder
gets pretty well squashed. Being composed of muscle, it tends to go
into spasm, similar to a spasm of the muscles of your leg. Since the
bladder is made of smooth muscle, you don't feel pain; what this
spasm does do, however, is diminish the holding capacity of the
bladder. It now simply holds less urine. The best way to get it back
to its normal size is to drink water and hold the water as long as
possible before urinating. In this way you are using the water itself
to re-stretch your bladder. It is very common for one of our female
patients to come to us after several weeks of drinking water and
complain that now she is "retaining" water, because she's not
going to the bathroom nearly as much as when she began. Yet,
when we have her measure the amount of water she is drinking
against the amount coming out, it is the same. She's not "retaining"
water at all; what has happened is that her urinary bladder has
dilated back to normal size and is holding more. As this happens,
those annoying trips to the bathroom are cut down and your water
drinking can continue without any problem.

YOUR CBO (CALORIE BURN-OUT) TIME
Each and every pound of your fat contains 3,500 calories. Do
you know what a calorie is? There's nothing really complicated
about it. A calorie is a unit of energy that comes from burning a
particular amount of fuel (food) for a particular length of time. It

stands to reason that if you can decrease the time, but keep the energy output the same, you will burn more calories, and your weight will come down faster. Because of the way the Nine-Day Wonder Diet is set up, this is precisely what will happen. We will discuss some of the specific mechanisms of this revolutionary concept as we guide you along the stages of the Plan. For now, just remember that you are on a plan that has been medically supervised by us, in use on people just like yourself. *They* did it. There's no reason in the world why *you* can't.

EMPTY CALORIES AND FULL CALORIES

Now that we've told you what a calorie is, and something about the guiding principle of the Nine-Day Wonder Diet—the CBO—we want to clear up a basic misconception about calories because there has been a great to-do about this in the popular press. You may have thought of a calorie being "empty" to the extent that it was something you could eat that wouldn't add weight. Nothing could be further from the truth. In point of fact there *are* food items that contain no calories, and we are going to be using them as part of your CBO. Beverages such as coffee, tea, Postum, carbonated water, mineral water and seltzer have no caloric value. Similarly, seasoning agents as celery salt, chives, cinnamon, dill, lemon juice, mint, onion, garlic, A-1 and Tabasco sauces have no calories to speak of. However, you can't live on these because their nutritive value is also nil, or pretty close to it.

Empty calories, for the overweight you, are worse than no calories. Like the foods above, they have no nutritive value, but they will be stored by your body as fat. They have nothing to offer in return for taking up space, nothing in the way of essential protein, fatty acids, minerals or vitamins to recommend them. They are really parasitic chemicals living off your body. You've opened the door and let them in. Where do they come from? Mainly from sugar, in all its forms, and hard cooking fat. It has been said that if sugar were discovered today it would be classified as a poison. No one in the world ever hungered for sugar. You may crave it from years of constant overuse, but recognize this craving as that of an addict. Both of us were tremendous sugar users for years. Neither

44

of us uses as much as a pinch of the stuff today. We're not saying this out of a sense of self-congratulation, but simply to show you that the addiction can be broken. If you can't or won't do this, no matter how many times you diet, you'll always get fat again. Remember the saying "You can't eat your cake and have it too"? *You* can. You're still carrying around the one you ate last week.

Cooking fats are the other main source of empty calories. Average ingestion of these by most people is about 500 calories per day (about 2 oz. of fat.) Now, remember, we're not talking about the fat that is included in milk, poultry, beef, lamb and lean pork, or the fat that you get from fruits and vegetables. Most of your empty calories come from meats like fatty pork, butter and margarine, though butter and margarine, while furnishing calories that are basically empty, do contribute a certain amount of vitamin A, so we utilize them in the Nine-Day Plan for that reason, and because they would be missed more than the others mentioned.

Cooking oils, however, are a different story. There is very little place for them in your life. Leave them on the TV screen with the people who get paid to say how great they are. They account for almost half the average individual's consumption of fat, and all they will do is make you fatter.

We don't want to tip the scale entirely against fat, though. First of all, it tastes good and that is a primary consideration of any food. Remember, we've already told you we are treating you as a person, not a piece of fat. Full calories, such as those mentioned above, contribute fat but add vitamins, minerals and other items essential to your health. And the fat you take in here will actually help you lose weight by making the foods you do eat more palatable, thereby keeping you on your plan. But fat from empty calories, which provide only weight and nothing else—these you can live without.

SAUCES AND CHEESES

We are going to allow you sauces and cheeses in moderation. That, of course, is a tricky word. Who decides what is a moderate amount? We do. Your Nine-Day Wonder Diet, while it includes a variety of possible alternatives, only allows you to shop around within pre-set limits. There is a saying among bariatricians—physicians who practice weight control—that the overweight patient cannot be given a choice. You'll choose wrongly every time. Look at yourself; haven't you proved it? It is your consistently wrong choices that have made you what you are today. "Give them a hand and they'll take off your entire arm" was the way one lecturer at a recent meeting put it. Any doctor who gives vague directions to an overweight patient is playing right into his hands. That is why you will find the Nine-Day Wonder Diet as specific as it is. Whatever leeway we have provided for you has been carefully calculated and redefined through our personal experience with patients who have not only been on the Nine-Day Plan alone, but have also combined it with the Food Intake Plan, shifting back and forth and losing, in the process, anywhere from thirty to over a hundred pounds. So don't be afraid to eat what we have provided; just remember that if it isn't on your Nine-Day Plan, you can't eat it at all. As far as you are concerned, it doesn't exist.

So ketchup and cocktail sauces may be used according to the amounts prescribed, as may horseradish, mustard and chili sauce. No mayonnaise. Vinegar is fine; you can use as much of that as you like. Be very careful about adding oil, however; no more than a quarter of a spoonful—remember what we had to say about empty calories. Don't forget lemon juice; it can be a real lifesaver when it comes to adding flavor to your food.

As for cheeses, step very gingerly here. Many cheeses contain quite a bit of salt as well as a goodly amount of fat. On the whole, skim-milk cheeses would be best; pot cheese, which doesn't have much fat content, would also be acceptable. Before adding any sort of cheese to your diet, even though we may allow it, get your cholesterol checked. This is especially necessary if, prior to going on the Nine-Day Plan, you've been on a cottage cheese diet of one form or another. It has been our experience that cottage cheese raises the blood cholesterol level faster than anything else. If your cholesterol is up, stay away from cheese, and probably also from eggs, at least until it goes down. Then watch the eggs and cheese very carefully.

EGGS AND FOWL

We've grouped these together since one comes from the other, though no one has decided in what order. You don't have to be chicken about eating eggs—provided you eat them only when and how your diet calls for them. It's hard to eat an egg slowly, but this is exactly how you must eat it or you will get no satiation from it and end up as hungry—or hungrier—than before you ate. There's a whole mystique about eggs. Rarely does one talk about eating an egg by itself. It always has to have company: ham and eggs, bacon and eggs, cheese omelet, eggs and potatoes, grits, toast, salad. Why? Because the usual fried egg slips past the palate so fast you don't even know it's been and gone. The best way to eat an egg is hard-boiled. This will furnish the most chewability and at least leave you with the impression that you've had some sort of a meal.

As for fowl, you can have any kind, but be careful about frying, particularly deep-fat frying. You can eat the skin; we do not consider this fat empty calories. Gnaw the bones (fowl is particularly good for this)—it's an activity that gives a great amount of oral satisfaction. Perhaps it is the primitive in us, but most people admit they really enjoy eating fowl more if they can pick up the pieces with their fingers. We've never been able to understand why this was frowned upon in the past, and why even now, at a dinner party, many people will hesitate to eat the last of the fowl with their fingers. An awful lot of good food gets wasted in this manner, and a lot more exuberance is expended on dessert that would have been better employed on bone-gnawing from the previous course. Overweight people in particular like to get as close to the food as possible, so don't worry about the etiquette of the situation. Just remind yourself that it's another good technique for weight loss.

SOME SUPPLEMENTAL BACKUPS

Multi-vitamin-mineral supplements. We urge you to take a good one daily. We provide these for our patients and you should get no less. This is not because we are at all worried about your becoming vitamin-deficient on the Nine-Day Wonder Diet, but we are dealing with all different types of individuals and we don't want even one of you to have the slightest qualm about lacking any of your necessary micronutrients. We won't recommend any particular brand name—you can see for yourself what the capsule contains by reading the label. We have found that there are some individuals who will cut down even more than we ask them to on the foods we supply; the vitamin-mineral supplement is even more important for them. It might be good to say right here that we do not advise cutting down in this manner. Not that it will do you any physical harm, but you will tend to think differently about the Plan; you'll expect to lose a lot more weight because you will be eating less, and this probably won't happen—or, if it does, not to the extent you might think it should. This will frustrate you and cast a pall of discontent over your diet. Better to do it just as we say. If you are not hungry and don't want to eat as much as you are offered, don't eat—but don't expect to see a lot more weight loss from that effect alone.

Methylcellulose. This is another good supplement that you can buy at your drugstore without a prescription. Methylcellulose is bulk, pure and simple. When you swallow it and drink water, the substance swells in your stomach, giving you a comfortable feeling of fullness. This will not only keep you from eating more than you should on your diet, it can be a considerable comfort on the fast days. Don't worry about becoming "addicted" to pills. There's nothing here that could possibly affect you in any way other than what you are taking it for. Basically the methylcellulose doesn't get into your body at all; it is never absorbed. But as it travels through your stomach and intestine it gives you the impression of having eaten well with none of the subsequent heartache (and heartburn) when you step on the scale. Be sure that you take enough so that you will get this effect: we recommend a minimum of 400 mg., and you can take this dosage three or four times a day. We have rarely used the methylcellulose in our practice with the Nine-Day Plan alone, but we have used it with our Food Intake Plan and with individuals who are combining both plans to lose a substantial amount of weight. It is a good aid and a reliable crutch that you can easily dispense with once you are able to use food alone as your basic weight-balancing mechanism.

48

Bran tablets. A lot has been written recently about the role of fiber in accelerating the weight-loss process, and we will have more to say about this in a later chapter. One of the advantages of an abundance of fiber in the diet is doing away with that usual plague of dieters: constipation. You can purchase bran tablets in most health-food stores; directions are on the bottle. Do not use the bran cereals instead. We will have a further discussion on cereals later on.

Protein hydrolosate liquid. We mention this here because in our office the subject always comes up when discussing fast days. It is not necessary for you to take any protein supplement during the time you will spend fasting on the Nine-Day Wonder Diet. We do not use this type of liquified protein ourselves; we did not use it when we lost our weight; we do not recommend it to other people. For this plan it is useless, particularly since, as it is a liquid, you get no satiation from it. You can't chew it, and the brands we have investigated have smelled and tasted pretty bad. However, if you think you need something like this to see you through your fast day, it probably won't hurt you. It is really meant for individuals who are on an extended fast, and if you are one of these you are certainly not on the Nine-Day Wonder Diet.

SPOT REDUCING

Among physicians in general, and among many of those doing weight control as well, the concept of "spot reducing"—getting your weight to come off those areas where its very presence was what induced you to go on a diet in the first place—is "faddism." Just what a fad is, we aren't sure. It appears to be something that is used successfully by somebody else. Remember: we said "successfully."

As a matter of fact, our office files are full of records of individuals—mainly women, but a number of men as well—who lost their inches just where they wanted to. Many of these people were on other diets when they came to us, had even lost weight on these plans, but were unhappy and disillusioned. Take the case of Shirley M.

Shirley was a large-boned woman, the type who can gain two or three pounds a week and never really notice it. Sound familiar? She came to us after being on a diet through which she'd lost fifty pounds. The trouble was, she was losing most of her weight in all the wrong places. But let us give you the story in Shirley's words:

"I keep losing inches in my breasts and upper body. My arms and my face are fine, but I can't afford any further bust loss—and just look at my hips and thighs. They're as fat as ever." With that she burst into tears. "I swear," she said, "I never thought I'd cry about my weight. Especially after losing fifty pounds. But I'd almost rather have it back again than look like this."

Fortunately, Shirley still had another twenty pounds to go before reaching normal weight. By placing her on two cycles of the Nine-Day Wonder Diet, alternated with two weeks of the Food Intake Plan, we were able to balance her CBO so that her weight began coming off where she wanted it—from her hips and thighs. When she got to normal weight and went on our Cycle Balancing Diet, she even put a little weight back on her bust while her thighs kept their newfound slimness.

Today she calls herself "a new person, freshly minted." A letter from her reads:

"I just can't thank you enough. Unfortunately, it isn't a final goal just to lose weight. It must be lost *from the right places* if any of us fat people are ever to feel like human beings again, feel like we are normally shaped. I know now, I'll never gain my weight back. I think that one of the reasons I did so before was because the fat never came off those parts of me I felt it should. Unfortunately, after dieting for years, no matter how much weight I lost, I still looked deformed."

We can't promise you that you'll look like the man or woman of your dreams—or someone else's dreams—when you finish with the Nine-Day Wonder Diet. We can promise you, however, that you have the best possible chance on this Plan to get your figure back to whatever it was before you put on your weight. If what you are fighting is the so-called middle-age spread, don't let that discourage you either. It isn't true that you haven't a chance because you're "over the hill." A hill, you know, can be climbed either way. As one lady recently told us: "I considered myself over the hill because of my weight and my age. They drove me there, *but I drove myself back.*"

Determination? You bet. That's the name of the game.

At the same time, even losing inches properly as you should on the Nine-Day Plan, it would be unrealistic of you to expect to come out with a whole new body. If you had wide hips or thighs before you got fat, you'll still have this characteristic when you get thin; body physique is mostly a family trait. But being fat makes these characteristics even more pronounced. Losing your unwanted inches may not make you a Venus de Milo or a Hercules but it can do even better. It can make you the individual You of just the right amount of flesh. That beats marble any day.

HOW THE NINE-DAY PLAN
REDUCES THOSE TROUBLESOME AREAS

You don't have to go on a special plan just to spot reduce. The standard Nine-Day Diet not only removes pounds, but you'll find those inches melting away as well—as evidenced by the surprising amounts of room you suddenly begin to find in your clothing. And, when you get to your normal weight, if there are still a few "bulgy" areas here and there, an extra cycle on the Wonder Diet may well slim them down, even though the amount of actual weight you lose may be minimal. The point is that you will see those extra inches go. Don't depend on your clothing to tell you, however. We ask you to measure yourself so that the evidence will be right there in your own calculations.

How does this work? Many people do not understand just how fat is stored in the body. They think it occurs only in soft "masses" or deposits, such as in the belly (abdomen) or breasts—and it is true that these are the main areas of storage. But fat is also stored within the muscle of the skeleton. Skeletal muscle is composed of strands rather loosely woven together. Excess fat can nest between these muscle strands to a greater or lesser extent. If these are the muscles of your thigh, the largest in the body, the extra bulk produced by this invading fat will make your thighs appear not only heavier but "bulgy"–even "lumpy"-looking, with an unpleasing, irregular character. The same holds true for the muscles of the buttocks or arms, and any other area where skeletal muscles normally protrude. But the fat that is stored in these areas only looks different from that stored in, say, the breasts, because of the nature of skeletal muscle. The fat is layered between these bundles of fibers, which are tied down at intervals.

Not long ago this "muscle fat" was given a new, more fashionable name: "cellulite." This is a totally made-up word, having no medical overtones despite the fact that it may aspire to them. At the same time, whatever you call it, getting rid of this muscle fat may be a more difficult process than losing fat elsewhere. You have probably been on diets where your weight came down all right, but those unsightly bulges didn't give an inch.

This should be no problem on the Nine-Day Wonder Diet. Your CBO has been calculated to utilize first the fat from your major deposits. As this diminishes, you should begin leaching out the fat from between the muscle fibers, all that lumpy host that has parked itself in these hard-to-get-at spaces. Notice that we have said "leaches out the fat." Nothing will happen to the muscle fibers themselves—nor would you want anything to occur here. Muscle is protein, and muscle tissue itself is never replaced. By exercising you can increase the size of a muscle—that is, make each individual fiber get larger—but you cannot increase the number of fibers.

The Nine-Day Plan won't affect your muscle fibers, your "lean mass" as it is called medically. But what you will find with the absorption of this muscle fat is a new feeling of "togetherness" within your body, an explosion of coordinated energy, as your skeletal muscle is finally liberated from the blanket of fat that has been keeping it from working at maximum efficiency.

Remember, you don't have to go on one plan to lose weight and on another to lose inches from those troublesome areas. The Nine-Day Plan offers you a method of losing both pounds *and* inches in a convenient, sensible and comfortable way. Who, even the heaviest of us, could ask for anything more?

YOU, TOO, CAN BE A SUCCESS

Madeline B. writes: "You've saved my life. My husband and I go to the Berkshires at least four times a year. I'm good for at least three extra pounds for the two days. The first time we went this year I took your Nine-Day Plan along which someone had given me. To my astonishment (I've been on plenty of diets) I found I not only had plenty to eat, I was *full*. The alcohol was just enough to allow for sociability; I made it last and found I didn't miss the extra two or three drinks I'd somehow always let the first one lead to. I ate normally and no one at our table knew I was on a diet. Such a relief not having to explain to strangers. I got on the scale when I got home feeling pretty scared—I felt so un-dieted—because I figured I'd gained *some* weight. To my astonishment I'd lost a pound and a half. Just from the first two days of the plan, even being away from home. When I weighed myself the following Sunday (after going to a wedding the previous day), I found I had lost a total of eight and a half pounds for the cycle. Nothing I've ever tried in my entire life has done this—including starvation. Thank you both for showing me a new way of living. You can bet that whenever my weight starts to go up, even a pound or two, it's back to a Nine-Day Cycle for me.''

And the head of a large corporation writes: ''I've been overweight for years and my doctors kept telling me I had to get it off. But my weekends would kill me. Lots of business dinners at the homes of clients or associates. For me to sit at the table constantly refusing what was served was downright humiliating. You've made it possible for me to feel like a normal human being again, entitled to enjoying my weekends without feeling I'm under some sort of taboo. The weekends were always what got me. By compensating for this—well, that makes your diet human and I could relate to it. Incidentally, I lost fifteen pounds on the first cycle alone.''

IF YOU GET SICK

Let's face it, being on the Nine-Day Wonder Diet isn't going to cure you of *everything*. You certainly are still liable to any sort of illness. You can get dizzy, catch a cold, get flushed, have a headache, get pregnant. All these things are possible. But please don't blame our plan. We've had women who've lost twelve to eighteen pounds in their first cycle of nine days, and then gotten pregnant. We have to assume that it was their *own* plan (or lack of) that brought that about.

Should you get a cold or a kidney stone or hemorrhoids, or almost any other medical ailment while you are on the Nine-Day Wonder Diet, don't go off it just because now you are "sick." Your real sickness is your overweight, and we are not telling you to do anything about it that will get you sick, or that will prevent you from recovering from any other illness that might occur simultaneously with your diet. Tell your family physician that you are on a plan for overweight; let him read this book. Chances are he's the one that has been on your back trying to get you to lose weight; he should be pleased to note that you have finally taken his advice.

If you follow our advice you may well join the long list of grateful people who have lost weight on this Plan. Two incidents from our office diary:

Yesterday Mary K. came in. She's come down from 227 to 145 pounds combining weeks of the Food Intake Plan with the Nine-Day Wonder Diet. This last nine days alone she's lost another eight pounds. She wants to get to 133. She'll make it. Before she left, we asked her how she feels compared to when she was fat. Her answer: "It's like a miracle the way these plans work. Things are different for me now. No matter what kind of a day it is, I can be happy. No matter who else is sad, I have something to be happy about. No one can ever take it away from me."

And JoAnn S.: "I was in a restaurant with my husband and a couple we hadn't seen since I'd lost the weight [she's lost 108 pounds to get to her present weight of 130] came over to say hello. They hemmed and hawed a little, and didn't seem to recognize me. Finally it dawned on me that they thought my husband was out with another woman, and were trying diplomatically to edge around to the subject when finally the woman broke through, saying, 'And how is your *wife*?' I've never been so pleased in my life."

We have hundreds of such stories in our office files, along with thousands of pictures of people who have lost a cumulative poundage of close to 200,000 pounds. You can be among them. Just don't get confused. There are a great number of diet plans around, all purporting to do the job. You may well ask, what makes ours different? We can answer that question like this:

All weight-loss plans deal with the same food elements: fats, proteins and carbohydrates. All deal with people. Our plan differs the way a pianist differs from a piano tuner. Both push down the same notes on the keyboard, but one makes noise, the other makes music. Our plan makes music: the sound of pounds falling off swiftly and painlessly.

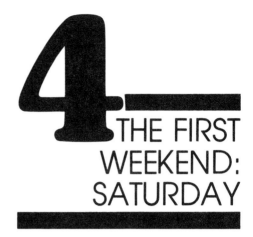

THE FIRST WEEKEND: SATURDAY

By now you should have an idea of the basic plan. We are at this point going to go right through each day with you so you'll know we're keeping an eye on you. Here is the basic meal plan for this day. Alternate menus will follow. Remember, it's a weekend, the time you usually manage to cheat on your diet. That's fine with us. Start "cheating" from whatever diet you've been following to this one. In this instance, cheating will help you lose weight.

THE MUST ITEMS FOR THIS DAY

These must items are not difficult, but they are essential to the success of your dieting plan. All instructions must be followed exactly.

1. You must drink eight 8-ounce glasses of water a day. If you wish, you may substitute seltzer or club soda, provided the club soda has only a minimum amount of salt. If drinking water isn't your cup of tea, don't substitute tea (or coffee) for it. You can, if you wish, add to your water the juice of one lemon and a little artificial sweetener.

2. Today you will eat three dried prunes, the kind with pits. They are to be divided through the day as follows: one at 10 A.M., 3 P.M. and one at 10 P.M. Do not substitute the de-pitted prunes. Once the prune goes, the pit will linger on, as a pacifier. The prunes supply potassium and thus help prevent you from getting leg cramps.

3. Exercise. You must do something to propel your skeleton beyond its routine daily movements. Your usual movements, strenuous as you may think they are, are routine to your body, which does not consider them exercise. Neither do we—because they do not get your pulse rate above normal. What, then, are we talking about? Running in place, for one thing. Try running in place for at least three minutes, three times a day. Take your pulse rate immediately following this activity. If it has not reached 120 beats per minute. you haven't exercised. If you have been ordered by your family doctor not to exercise, or if you cannot do any form of exercise so strenuous as running, you can still walk. Walk around the block for three minutes as briskly as you can and then check your pulse rate. Keep a record of it in your logbook. If you persist, even taking your exercise a little at a time, you will eventually get your pulse rate up to 120. That's when you begin to do yourself some good.

Now, here we go. As you know, the Nine-Day Wonder Diet starts on a Saturday and ends the following Sunday, encompassing two weekends and the days between. At the end of this time you should be between eight and twelve pounds lighter IF you do exactly as we have instructed you. If you do not lose this much weight, do not be discouraged. Chances are you "goofed" somewhere along the way but, unless you goofed pretty badly, you still will have lost *some* weight. The best thing for you to do is read through the first portion of this book, reviewing especially Chapter 2, and start another cycle when a convenient Saturday comes along. One thing about a cyclical plan is very reassuring: there's always another cycle and the very next one may be your turn to get on.

Breakfast

The time you eat is very important. Get up around eight o'clock and either run in place for three minutes or take a brisk walk. Do not have anything, even water, at this time. By eight-thirty you should be at the breakfast table. Do *not* eat later than nine o'clock—that is, do not start your meal any later than that. If you haven't made it to breakfast between 8:30 and 9, don't eat. Just skip breakfast; it won't kill you.* We have calculated your CBO and if you overlap meal zones you won't lose the weight you should. So if you decide that you'd rather sleep late on a Saturday or Sunday morning, that's fine with us. You will then forget about breakfast entirely and start a new CBO with lunch.

BASIC MENU: Day 1

¼ *canteloupe*

½ *bagel* with either a low-calorie jelly or butter or margarine on it (no more than ½ teaspoon).

1 egg, any style. (It is best if you take it closer to the hard than the oversoft. In other words, less coddled, more poached. Best is hard-boiled.

You may use margarine or butter for frying, but no more than ½ teaspoon.

Beverages: Coffee or tea. Two teaspoons of regular milk may be used. No sugar. Use all artificial sweeteners carefully; they are salts, usually sodium saccharide, and will, if overused, inhibit your weight loss.

SUBSTITUTIONS: For the canteloupe: ⅛ honeydew melon or 1 small orange, but not orange juice.

For the bagel: ½ slice rye or whole-wheat toast. Butter or margarine may be used as described.

For milk: any of the milk substitutes such as Coffeemate or skim milk.

Lunch

This meal must be eaten between 12:30 and 1:30 P.M. If you cannot eat between those times, or if you are not hungry then, skip lunch entirely; eating is not mandatory on the Nine-Day Plan. But if you do skip lunch, remember that you will have nothing to eat until dinner. It's not all that bad; we've done it. You can get by very nicely with your water intake—and remember, you *are* eating. Your body is nibbling at those fat deposits, eating internally, eating all the time. That's the only way you get rid of excess weight: by having your body eat it up.

* Of course, if you're one of those people who gets up at noon and goes to sleep in the small hours, simply modify the schedule, keeping the same time-span between meals.

BASIC MENU: Day 1

4 oz. tomato juice

Salad: to make 3 cups use the following raw vegetables in any proportion you choose: lettuce, celery, cauliflower, spinach, cabbage, cucumber, asparagus, broccoli, mushrooms.

Spices: You may use any combination of the following in a quantity of your choice: vinegar, lemon juice, garlic, herbs, mustard, onion, horseradish, olive oil (take it easy here), pepper, salt substitute if necessary. As usual, WATCH THE SALT. Use it sparingly, if at all.

Cheese: You may add 3 oz. of shredded Swiss cheese to the salad.

Beverages: Coffee, tea or 8 oz. nonsugared soda. And, of course, water.

SUBSTITUTIONS: For the juice you may substitute 4 oz. of V-8 or unsweetened pineapple juice. You may not want juice at all; in that case substitute 1 medium tomato.

For the cheese: 3 oz. of Mozzarella or Feta cheese may be used instead of the Swiss.

Dinner

As with the two previous meals, there is a strict time for eating dinner. It should be eaten between 6:30 and 7:30 P.M. There is no relationship between the time you eat dinner and the time you go to bed.

BASIC MENU: Day 1

Pre-dinner cocktail: 1 oz. of any liquor of your choice. Refer to the previously noted caloric table regarding alcohol. Whatever you drink, make it last. You may have your drink on the rocks with water or with club soda—or straight if you really need a quick pick-me-up to celebrate your having gotten through the day thus far. Please do not misunderstand us. Many of our patients have made the mistake of assuming they *had* to have a drink, whether they wanted to or not. Having alcohol is by no means mandatory; if you don't want a drink, by all means leave it. On the other hand, don't have more than one on the happy assumption that you are drinking up someone else's refusal.

1 cup clear broth or bouillon.

5 oz. meat—that is, beef, lamb or veal. No pork whatsoever is allowed today. How do you prepare these dishes? However you best like them; we ask only that you do not deep-fat fry or bread this meat.

1 cup vegetables. A choice of two of the following either cooked or raw: summer squash, spinach, green beans, onions, cabbage, cauliflower, celery, eggplant or broccoli. You may use ½ teaspoon margarine or butter in the cooking.

Dessert: ½ cup any berries with ⅓ cup milk or cream.

Beverages: Coffee or tea.

Substitutions: You may substitute for both vegetables ½ cup home-fried or oven-broiled potatoes with 1 tablespoon oil. For the bouillon, you may substitute ½ cup asparagus soup.

SNACKING, NOT SNEAKING

You may feel that you have to eat something between meals. If this urge becomes so pressing that you can't resist it, we would rather have you turn to the following lists rather than go off on your own. Remember, this will slow down your CBO, though you will still lose weight, provided that you stay with the portions provided. If you exceed them, you may disrupt your entire Cycle. Even with a snack it is necessary to follow the eating behavior you should be putting into effect with your scheduled meals: eat slowly, sit down, chew well, pay attention to what you are eating rather than to what you are watching, reading or saying. And above all remember: a snack is anything you put into your mouth that fills you up and that will put as little weight on you as possible by disrupting your CBO as little as possible. There is a difference between a Snack and a Sneak. A Sneak is going for those foods that are not on the Plan, that you know *will* add to your weight, that have always betrayed you before and that are tremendous sources of empty calories. Any amount of such items, regardless how small ("I only ate a little" is the swansong of many a diet) will not only dampen your CBO but will likely extinguish it for the next twenty-four hours or more, depending on the quantity you eat. It's easy not to Sneak. Each time you don't do it makes it easier not to do it the next time, and finally you're doing no Sneaking and not even patting yourself on the back for it. At that point sensible eating will have become a way of life. For Snacking, not Sneaking, look at the following lists. The first contains items that have no calories at all to speak of, though a few of them do contain salt and you must be aware of this; we have placed an asterisk next to these foods. This doesn't mean you can't use them; just don't choose them if you've a condition that will be aggravated by even a small amount of salt. If you are a woman and you are premenstrual, you should be wary of any intake of salt at this time. If you are a man or a woman with high blood pressure or severe water retention, the same holds true and you should work around these items. Here they are:

FOOD ITEMS THAT CONTAIN NO CALORIES (Snack List #1)

Beverages:

   Black Coffee. (You may use two teaspoons of skim milk or even whole milk without disturbing your CBO, provided that you drink no more than three cups a day this way.) You can drink as much black coffee as you wish. Caffeine helps fight hunger and will help remove excess water from your system.

   Postum. The same holds true here as for coffee.

   Tea. The same holds true here as for coffee. You cannot add all these items together—three cups of any with milk is the limit.

   Carbonated water. * Some of these that you get in the store may contain higher percentages of salt than others. Compare labels.

   Mineral water. Either the natural or artificial variety is equally good.

   Seltzer water. * This may contain a minimal amount of salt, but you can substitute it for almost half your water if you desire. Many people find it more palatable than plain drinking water.

   Diet sodas. * Salt here is found in compounds such as sodium citrate and sodium carbonate. You must limit yourself to no more than 8 oz. of diet soda daily. We also caution you about the dye contained in many of them. It would probably be better for your stomach to drink the clear diet sodas rather than those containing dye.

Sugar Substitutes:

Saccharine

Sucaryl or Sweet 'n Low

Seasoning Agents

Chopped celery, 1 stalk. The idea is to use this as a seasoning agent with some of the items on Snack List #2.

Chives (as a seasoning to be used with selected items on Snack List #2).

Cinnamon

Dill

Monosodium glutamate

Lemon juice (or sections or slices. Very refreshing once you get used to it).

Lime. The same here as with lemon. We recommend learning to nibble at these particular citrus fruits, skin and all—though lime skin is more difficult to chew than lemon. You'll be surprised to find how refreshing lemon skin can be, and here's a useful trick to apply with your cocktail ration. If you are choosing a martini, get it with a number of "twists" and nibble these between sips. This makes a built-in hors d'oeuvre that is suitable for almost any other drink as well. This little ploy may be all you need to keep you from reaching for the dangerous substances on the snack tray. No olives in the martini, incidentally.

Mint. You can put fresh mint in your cocktail, even in your water if you require some flavoring, and you can nibble it for refreshment as with the lemon peel. Dried mint, of course, would be used as a seasoning.

Mustard.

Onion powder.

Onion slices. Eat these raw, not cooked.

Paprika.

Pepper. All varieties are acceptable, especially Lawry's Seasoned Pepper. This category also includes the peppers from your garden—red, green, hot or bell. You may eat up to ½ bell pepper as a snack or one small sample of the other varieties.

Pimento.

Salt substitutes. These have various tastes and you will have to shop around to find the one that suits you. Don't be discouraged if some that you try are less than satisfactory. Keep looking for the one you feel you can live with; it's there, someplace. Our own choice is Adolph's.

Sauces. * In chapter 5 we give you the recipes for a number of these as well as for some spreads. Worcestershire, A-1 and Tabasco are some good commercial sauces you may use. Again, watch the salt.

Spices. Cider, wine or artificial vinegar are all fine and will give you a good base for salad dressing. (See Chapter 5 for salad dressing instructions.)

Garlic. Fresh clove garlic or garlic powder are fine, but garlic salt should be avoided, as previously noted.

Pickles. Remember, the pickling process utilizes a lot of salt so, once again, be wary. In extreme moderation you can use dill pickles, bread and butter, cucumber or sour pickles. You can use relish as well as pickled onions.

Soups

Bouillon
Clear soups with the fat skimmed off
Consommés
Jellied consommé
Tomato bouillon

Delicacies

Prunes. Only on the days indicated.
Apricots. Only on the days indicated.
Cranberry sauce. A one-inch slice only.
Rhubarb. (unsweetened)

FOOD ITEMS THAT CONTAIN MINIMAL CALORIES (Snack List #2)

These are all vegetables, best eaten raw. We have calculated them as snacks based on a standard portion of ½ cup whether mixed or single. Remember, these are meant to be snacks, not a meal.

Asparagus (either fresh or canned stalks)

String Beans. These may be boiled or served cold with seasonings from Snack List #1. This makes a delicious, very low-calorie snack.

Beet greens. Serve like string beans.

Cauliflower. Serve raw or boiled, with seasoning or plain.

Celery

Cucumber

Endive

Escarole

Lettuce

Mushrooms

Parsley

Pepper

Pickles. Apply the same cautions as with Snack List #1.

Radishes

Spinach. Serve plain, not creamed.

Squash

If you are going to snack—and remember, it is not mandatory—the best time to do it is before five o'clock in the evening. *Never snack after that time,* as you will disrupt your CBO. We have furnished you on occasion with a piece of fruit prior to bed, but these are specific instances on specific menus. You cannot join the portions of one day's menu to another; if the piece of fruit you want doesn't occur on the day's menu you are on, don't eat it. Don't start thinking, "It's such a small thing...what difference does it make...who will know?" It's a big thing as far as your CBO is concerned. The difference it makes could be considerable for your weight loss. And as to "who will know?"—*you* will know. As far as we are concerned, *you* are the most important person on your diet. But should you go off it temporarily, don't worry and, above all, don't feel guilty. Just go right back on and pick up where you left off. There are enough defeating incidents in life for all of us without adding dieting to the list. We can tell you that your Nine-Day-

Wonder Diet is never defeating. Even if you go on it only part way, you'll still lose weight.

But why go on it part way when the whole thing is so easy to do? You have accomplished the first weekend with little if any difficulty and a great feeling of accomplishment. Or, if you haven't yet begun, start now,. Take the first steps on the road to an amazing success. We offer you proved success in an area in which most people—perhaps even you—have failed over and over. We ask of you only a small amount of your personal cooperation to be that healthier, happier slimmed down You of your dreams.

ALTERNATE TIMES OF EATING

Since this is a Saturday, and Saturday night is a routine "going out" occasion for many people, you can tailor your diet to this activity if necessary, at least for the time spans of this day. But don't ad lib this; follow the procedure here laid down regarding the time, and don't do this at the last moment. You must know in advance what your plans are; if something comes up suddenly, you must follow the basic mealtimes. If you intend to be out late Saturday night—or are going to be entertaining at home and have planned dinner for a later hour than usual—eat breakfast that morning no earlier than ten o'clock, no later than eleven. Lunch should be timed between 3 and 4, and dinner between 8 and 9:30. You may want to save your one ounce of alcohol for later that night or, if there are to be cocktails at a prearranged time, you could have it then. This alternate meal-zoning schedule should help you get through the evening more comfortably.

Before retiring on Saturday night you may have a snack of one apple or one pear, and you can make it the biggest you can find. Eat it slowly; this will make it seem even bigger.

ALTERNATE MENUS

You may utilize these instead of the basic menu discussed above; all include the one-ounce drink of alcohol if you want it. While there may appear to be more to eat on some of these alternates than on others, that is because you are an individual and are entitled to have a little more if that is what it will take to truly satisfy you. At the same

65

time, we have calculated the CBO on all of these and, whichever you choose, you will be on the road to taking off pounds and inches with a rapidity that will astonish you. Make no substitutions whatsoever on these alternate menus. You really shouldn't even want to. Look them over; you'll be amazed at how many creative, healthful dishes are available for you to start this pleasant, easy program.

ALTERNATE MENU #1: Meat Loaf

Breakfast   2 oz. canned salmon (drain oil, no dressing)
        2 lettuce leaves (small)
        1 slice whole-wheat toast
        ½ cup citrus fruit
        coffee or tea

Lunch   2 oz. cottage cheese
        3 oz. turkey
        2 slices tomato with ½ teaspoon French dressing
        1 slice whole-wheat bread
        coffee or tea

Dinner   4 oz. meat loaf
        ½ baked potato, small
        1 teaspoon Wesson oil
        ½ cup creamed spinach
        4 oz. fruit in season

Alternate Menu #2: Steak

Breakfast   1 sliced orange
        ½ cup bran cereal with ½ glass skim milk
        1 egg, hard-boiled
        coffee or tea

Lunch   1 cup shrimp salad
        ½ teaspoon diet salad dressing or 1 teaspoon shrimp cocktail sauce
        1 slice whole-wheat bread
        ½ cup buttermilk

Dinner   1 cup bouillon
        4 oz. steak (rare, medium or well done)
        ½ cup spinach, kale or mustard greens

½ cup Jello with ½ fruit cup
1 glass skim milk or coffee or tea

Alternate Menu #3: Veal Fricassee

Breakfast 2 oz. unsweetened pineapple juice
½ cup oatmeal with ½ cup milk
coffee, tea

Lunch ½ cup cottage cheese
2 lettuce leaves
1 slice melba toast
½ sliced orange
coffee, tea

Dinner 4 oz. Veal fricassee
carrots and celery, cooked, ½ cup each
1 small lettuce wedge with lemon juice
½ cup citrus fruit
1 slice whole-wheat bread
coffee or tea

Alternate Menu #4: Chopped meat

Breakfast ½ grapefruit
3 oz. broiled kippers
½ cup oatmeal with 2 tablespoons skimmed milk
coffee, tea

Lunch 2 eggs, fried in Teflon pan
1 slice whole-wheat bread with ½ teaspoon butter
coffee, tea

Dinner 4 oz. tomato juice
4 oz. hamburger—rare, medium or well done
1 small roll
½ cup coleslaw (vinegar dressing)
½ cup Jello
coffee, tea

Alternate Menu #5: London Broil

Breakfast 1 sliced orange
½ cup bran cereal
4 oz. cottage cheese

1 slice whole-wheat toast
coffee, tea

Lunch ½ cup fresh melon balls

4 oz. tuna fish salad (you may use ½ tablespoon mayonnaise)

2 slices large tomato

½ cup Jello

coffee, tea

Dinner 4 oz. London broil or liver

½ cup asparagus

celery, carrot sticks, green pepper rings

½ citrus fruit cup

coffee, tea

1 cup skimmed milk when desired

Alternate Menu #6: Veal Piccata

Breakfast ½ cup any berries

½ cup any dry cereal

1 glass skimmed milk

coffee, tea

Lunch 3 oz. sliced cold chicken

lettuce, celery, cucumber, radish to make 1½ cups

1 slice whole-wheat bread

½ sliced orange

coffee, tea

Dinner Veal piccata

tossed salad: 1 cup lettuce, onion, mushrooms, two slices of tomato, garlic powder

1 tablespoon diet dressing, any kind

½ cup lemon sherbet

coffee, tea

Alternate Menu #7: Lamb Goulash

Breakfast ½ cup unsweetened grapefruit sections

1 slice whole-wheat bread

4 oz. cottage cheese

1 egg fried in Teflon pan

68

1 teaspoon unsweetened marmalade
coffee, tea

Lunch 2 oz. vegetable juice
salad: 2 cups sliced tomato, scallions, mushrooms, parsley
2 tablespoons wine vinegar
1 slice whole-wheat bread
½ teaspoon butter or margarine
coffee, tea

Dinner 2 oz. tomato juice
1 small baked potato
lamb goulash
1 teaspoon unsweetened mint jelly
½ cup green salad with lemon oil
1 cup Jello
coffee, tea

Alternate Menu #8: Rib Lamb Chops

Breakfast ½ cup orange juice
½ cup shredded wheat
½ cup skimmed milk
coffee, tea

Lunch 1 fruit cup
1 slice whole-wheat bread with 1 teaspoon unsweetened
jam
coffee, tea

Dinner 1 cup tomato soup
lettuce wedge with lemon
lamb chop (grilled or broiled; if necessary you may have
two)
1 small baked potato
coffee, tea

Alternate Menu #9: Irish Stew

Breakfast ½ cup unsweetened orange or grapefruit juice
1 slice whole-wheat toast with unsweetened jam OR ½
teaspoon butter or margarine
1 poached egg
coffee, tea

Lunch ½ cup fresh strawberries
1 glass skim milk
small can tuna fish with lemon juice
coffee, tea
Dinner 1 cup clear soup
Irish Stew—using either lamb or veal
½ cup baked noodles with 1 tablespoon cottage cheese
coffee, tea

Recipes for Saturday, Day 1

1. Meat Loaf

½ lb. ground beef	2 teaspoons Lawry's Seasoned
½ lb. ground veal	Pepper
½ cup bread crumbs	½ teaspoon Ehler's Garlic
2 eggs, beaten	Powder
⅛ teaspoon paprika	¼ teaspoon dry mustard
½ cup chopped onion	⅛ teaspoon black pepper

Mix the two meats well with the bread crumbs. Add eggs after beating. Stir in onions and other seasonings, put in finely buttered pan, bake at 350 degrees for approximately 1 hour. Serves 5.

2. Steak

Lawry's seasoned pepper	tenderloin beef with fat
Ehler's Garlic Powder	trimmed off
sirloin, club, porterhouse or	black pepper, onions, mushrooms

Steak may be cooked to any degree you like it as long as it is broiled: rare, medium or well done—it makes no difference. When you remove it from the oven, drain excess fat from the meat. Sprinkle on condiments prior to broiling, add onions and mushrooms and serve.

3. Veal Fricassee

2 lbs. boneless veal	3 onions
2 tablespoons margarine	2 tablespoons chopped parsley
1 tsp. Ehler's Seasoned Peppei	2 cups cooked rice
4 carrots	

Make sure meat is dry; pat slices with paper towel. Cut into pieces

70

about 1 inch thick and brown in small amount of margarine. Sprinkle Ehler's Pepper on meat, add water to cover. Simmer about an hour, until meat is tender. Add vegetables 30 minutes before meat is ready; stir all together over high heat to boiling. Pour over rice and serve. Serves 5.

4. Chopped meat

1 ½ lbs. ground beef chuck
1 egg
1 teaspoon Ehler's Seasoned
  Pepper
½ cup chopped onion

black pepper
3 tablespoons Wesson oil
parsley
2 tablespoons ketchup or Heinz
  tomato soup.

For best flavor meat should be freshly cut and ground only one time. Mix well with egg and seasonings. Add the onions and ketchup. Heat oil very hot while making patties; place patties in pan and brown each side. Use spatula to turn, as the patties may easily break apart if you use a fork. Cook through to your taste. Drain excess oil (patties should be drained on paper towel), serve with sprinkling of parsley. You may add raw onion if desired. Another variation: Instead of ketchup or Heinz tomato soup, mix in half a can of Heinz Mushroom soup. Serves 5.

5. London Broil

A 2- to 3-pound flank steak is an excellent piece of meat if prepared properly. The trick here is in the carving and the broiling. If you do not like your meat rare, stay away from this one, as flank steak gets very tough if cooked any other way. Broil right up next to the heat, about five minutes on each side. Flavor the meat with Seasoned Pepper, a dash of black pepper and 1 teaspoon margarine spread on each side. When carving, slice diagonally across the grain. This is a great favorite among our patients when done right.

6. Veal Piccata

2 to 3 lbs. veal slices, pounded
  very thin
lemon juice
Ehler's Garlic Powder

Lawry's Seasoned Pepper
salt substitute
parsley
flour

71

Make certain the meat is as thin as you can get it; these slices should be absolutely free of bone. Make a thin paste of flour and water; add to it the seasonings. In a pan place two tablespoons Wesson oil (we have found this oil to have the smallest amount of additives) and heat it until very hot. Dip the meat into the flour paste, then fry in oil. Use the minimum of flour. Serve piping hot garnished with parsley and plenty of lemon juice. Serves 5.

7. Lamb (or Veal) Goulash

1 lb. lamb (shoulder or shank)
2 tablespoons Wesson oil
Salt substitute and Lawry's Sea-
    soned Pepper
dried ground ginger

flour
1½ cups beef or chicken stock
1 clove garlic or Ehler's powder
1 tablespoon sherry

Heat the oil well in a large skillet and cut your meat into pieces about 1 inch in diameter. Season with Lawry's Pepper and the ginger. Dip each piece into the flour and make sure it is completely covered. Then brown the meat in the hot oil, add the stock and the garlic. (The clove, of course, needn't be crushed. You may, if you wish, substitute the garlic powder.) Cook about 1 hour or bake in oven at 325 degrees for about the same length of time. Add sherry. Remove garlic clove, if whole, before adding wine; drain off excess fat with spoon before serving. This goes well on a bed of rice, of which you may have two tablespoons on your plate. Serves 4.

8. Rib Lamb Chops

These should be broiled similarly to the broiled steak previously described. Fresh mint is a useful garnish here instead of parsley. Occasionally, you may add unsweetened pineapple slices. While we have nothing against pan-broiled chops, most people fail to remove enough of the fat that accumulates in most pan broiling. If you are going to try pan broiling, your meat should not be more than ½-inch thick and quite lean. Season with Lawry's Seasoned Pepper and Ehler's Garlic Powder.

9. Irish Stew

1 ½ lb. lamb shoulder	black pepper
flour	5 medium potatoes
3 tablespoons butter	2 celery stalks
water	5 carrots
2 teaspoons Lawry's Seasoned Pepper	1 onion

Cut the meat into stew-sized pieces; take the skin off the potatoes and cut them into pieces about 1 inch cubed. Make sure the meat is dry; roll the pieces in flour; brown well in the hot butter. Add about 1 cup of water; let simmer for an hour, then add condiments and vegetables and another 1 to 2 cups of boiling water. In about thirty minutes everything should be evenly tender. You may add 1 tablespoon of sherry or any other cooking wine five or ten minutes before serving. Serves 5.

WINE

You will note that we have allowed you to cook with wine—this is in addition to your one ounce of alcohol predinner drink. This does not mean that you can drink a glass of wine, as in the old recipe: Take three ounces of chopped meat, add one egg and pour two ounces of wine into the chef. It is not exactly the same if the wine goes into you or into the food. Alcohol is very volatile, and it will mostly cook out of the food, leaving only the flavor of the grape behind to nudge your palate. Remember that all alcohol—and this includes wine—is a source of empty calories: it has no more amino acids, vitamins or minerals than does sugar. At the same time, you didn't gain all that weight from just one drink, so enjoy it.

One question always comes up: Is it better to have your drink "on the rocks" or mixed with water or club soda? As long as you only have one, it doesn't matter; you will get the same amount of alcohol either way. However, to make your drink last longer, we advise diluting it. Be careful, though, that what you use to dilute it (orange or pineapple juice, sugared mixes) doesn't contain more calories than the alcohol. It's best to stick to water or club soda (or seltzer if you can get it) to mix with your alcohol. As for what kind of alcohol is best on this Plan: bourbon, scotch, vodka, you name it. But only name it once.

MILK AND BUTTERMILK

The caloric values of whole or skimmed milk are fairly constant. One cup of whole cow's milk (eight ounces) equals 165 calories, while the same amount of skim, nonfat milk equals 90 calories. The same amount of buttermilk also comes to 90 calories, provided you get the correct kind of buttermilk. We have allowed you buttermilk on the Nine-Day-Plan. You will find it in the Saturday Diet and you will find it in recipes for the other days. *Caution:* Read the label on the buttermilk bottle or container. Only if it is labeled "skimmed milk buttermilk" or "nonfat buttermilk" is it what you are looking for. If it is not so labeled, consider it about 120 calories per eight-ounce cup and beware of it. A number of our patients have come to grief in exactly this situation, and then were quite puzzled as to why they didn't lose the proper amount of weight on the Plan. Even skim-milk buttermilk varies a little per container, but it averages out to around 85-90 calories per cup. It is surprising to many people to find that skim milk has the same amount of calories as buttermilk and that whole milk has almost twice as many.

As for the milk in your coffee or tea, limit yourself to two teaspoons of whole milk if you drink only three or four cups of these beverages a day. If you are a heavy coffee or tea drinker—anywhere from eight cups on up—limit yourself to one teaspoonful of skim milk per cup. Milk products such as cheese, cream, and so on are outlawed except where specifically indicated. Keep in mind that this is for one cycle—nine days—only. If all you have is ten pounds to lose, chances are that you will be able to go back to an eating plan that will include these missing items...so long as you understand that if you don't use the top of your head before you use the bottom section, you will get fat all over again.

GUM CHEWING

You can chew all the gum you want between meals, provided it is sugarless gum. Like smoking, chewing involves mouth satisfaction and pacifying. You don't swallow the gum; it is just utilized to keep your jaws moving and to fool your mouth into thinking that it is full. Where you have time between meals, sugarless gum is an ideal "snack."

Today, Saturday You Will Drink 2 oz. Tomato Juice ½ Hr. Before Each Meal

Day 1 of your Nine Day Wonder Diet calls for you to drink two ounces of tomato juice three times a day. It is critical that you not only do this, but do it at the proper time. This does not substitute for the water drinking that you will be doing in any event, every day. The main reason for the tomato juice is that your CBO is increased by drinking it. We aren't trying to impute mysterious properties to the tomato in particular. Other foods work as well—if combined with the specific foods on the Nine-Day Plan. We have selected tomato juice for this first day since it is a convenient item, has the amount of calories we want (approximately ten), is not expensive and most people like it. If you are one who does not, or if for some reason you cannot ingest tomatoes, you may substitute one ounce of orange-grapefruit juice (twelve calories.) Do not make the mistake of substituting any of the orange-flavored *drinks*. We are talking only about *juice* here.

THE SPECIFIC DYNAMIC ACTION OF FOODS

Why does this work on your CBO? Your calorie burn-out—which is how fat is lost from your body—is based on a process referred to as the "specific dynamic action of foods." This is another way of saying that food itself, or at least certain foods, can cause an increase in body metabolism (calorie burn-out) and are not stored as fat. Perhaps this is the reason why your thin friends can eat and eat and eat and never put on a pound: their calorie burn-out is immense. For many years there has been a theory in medicine that the overweight individual has some sort of defect in his or her mechanism relating to this specific dynamic action. Putting it more simply, your calorie burn-out may either be malfunctioning or entirely absent, leaving whatever *you* eat to be stored as fat. This despite the fact that you, as an overweight person, expend more energy doing the same amount of work as a thin person may.

Based on this theory we came up with the idea of the Calorie Burn-Out: that is, that small amounts of extra calories, if combined with an overall weight-loss system and taken at the proper times with the proper foods, might well act as stimulators to provoke the body to mobilize additional calories from stored fat and thereby allow this specific dynamic action to take place.

We don't want to bore you with too much theory. Suffice it to say that in practice not only did our patients lose weight, but they acquired a sense of well-being that most of them claimed not to have experienced since they were in high school. "I was even fat in high school," one businessman told us rather shamefacedly. "I don't know when I've ever felt so effective." This was after two cycles of the Nine-Day Plan. You can feel the same way.

In addition, the juice will get rid of some of the bland taste you may have in your mouth from the water you've been drinking. The small amount of salt present in the juice will refresh your taste buds. It also provides you with natural vitamin C.

SWIFT RESULTS FROM CALORIE BURN-OUT IF...

You must follow all instructions precisely. You must do everything we tell you in the order that we have presented your day. There are no shortcuts on the Nine-Day Diet. The Plan itself is short enough and, if you follow it, will cut off a lot of time wasted on other plans. A word of warning: When you start one of the alternate menus, you must follow through that entire day. In other words, you can't take a lunch from one, a breakfast from another, a dinner from a third. We have certainly provided you with enough variety to enable you to pick and choose without ad libbing out of perversity or carelessness. Either way it will end up sheer foolishness. Each day has been carefully balanced by us according to your proper CBO; if you mix up the meals you'll end up eating your heart out.

On the other hand, if you follow your Nine-Day Plan to the letter, you will find that not only are you losing weight faster than you ever believed possible, not only are you not hungry, but you are enjoying the taste of food possibly for the first time in your life.

5.
THE FIRST WEEKEND: SUNDAY

You probably feel pretty good this morning. You've every reason to. You came through yesterday without the need to go off your diet and you don't have the guilty feeling that you may have woken up with in the past, on Sundays, thinking about how "bad" you were with food and drink the night before. Surprisingly, not only weren't you hungry, but you had more energy than you can remember having in the past—and you weren't even tempted to go off the Plan. This is a major reason for starting on a Saturday, when your resolve is fresh and the Plan has not become a routine. The truth of the matter is that this diet will never become routine and you can wake up every morning—not only while you are on the Nine-Day Wonder Diet, but every morning for the rest of your life—feeling this good and this effective. Instead of poisoning yourself with food, you are using it as the basic drug to fight overeating. Why hasn't anyone ever told you about this before? Well, we're telling it to you now, and better late than never. Our patients feel the same way. "Why didn't anyone ever tell me it was this easy?" one woman exclaimed to us after losing twelve pounds in a little less than nine days. "I've been dieting all my life and all I've done is pick one from column A and one from column B...and when I wasn't hungry the diets *made* me eat. This one is so reasonable."

Well, you're going to find that out for yourself. But meanwhile, you've still got eight days to go and a lot of adventure, surprise and weight loss yet to come. Let's see what Sunday will bring.

GET INTO YOUR EXERCISE ROUTINE THIS DAY

We haven't really pushed you into exercising so far. We more or less left it up to you yesterday, but Sunday is a good day to really get your exercise options in order. Usually it is a restful day and even if later on you have company, the morning should be your own.

As we said earlier in this book, we do not recommend strenuous exercises for overweight people. In our practice we treat individuals who weigh over four hundred pounds; for them a jog around the block could be fatal. In addition, most people—whether overweight or not—find exercise boring. That's all right. We're going to break up your exercise into three daily periods. It has been found that the first three to five minutes of exercise are the most productive from the standpoint of calorie loss; and this may well be because most people get tired of the exercise shortly after that point and begin to waver from the set pattern. Since the first three to five minutes are the enthusiastic time, we want to pack all that enthusiasm of yours into three minutes and then stop. Chances are, that will make you even more enthusiastic. When you stop, stop abruptly; don't bother tapering off. And start abruptly, too; as you know, most of your warm up time before doing exercise is really a way of putting off the actual physical activity that burns up calories. So make up your mind to do it, finish the three minutes and quit. All quite painless. But you must do this three times a day without fail. You don't have to do the same exercise for each of the three intervals, but you must do one of them each time. The first time you forget, you've set your entire weight-loss plan back two days. The first time you forget, it makes it that much easier to forget the following interval. And before you know it, you're right back where you were—getting your exercise by talking about exercising. We found that the doing of these exercises, *this often,* is more important than the specific exercises you do. Let's look at a few:

Running in place. Very easy. There's no outdoor clothing involved and no preparation. You can do it while watching TV or even while reading a book. Don't worry about looking foolish; no one is there to see and, if members of your family do come in, they should be the last ones to discourage you. Now, though we've encouraged you to do other things while running in place, don't get so involved, in, say, watching television or reading that you slow down your physical activity. Check your pulse every so often. Your pulse rate must be above 120 beats per minute or your exercising is that in name only. Get some sort of timer that will tell you when three minutes are up. Such a device is strictly unprejudiced. It will remember the time you started and there won't be any question about when the time is over. REMEMBER: THREE MINUTES, THREE TIMES A DAY.

Jogging. We like to think of this as "plodding." It is our strong feeling that plodding is safer than jogging. Too many individuals jog as though they were practicing for the Olympics. Before they know it, their jogging has become actual running. If you get carried away with your jogging in this manner, one of these days you may get literally carried away. So plod, don't run. Don't show off to yourself how good you are. Other than this, jogging is an easy exercise to do for three minutes. You can jog in just about any weather if you dress for it. Your pulse should get to 120; you needn't go above this. Jogging for a minute and a half with a pulse at 200 isn't better than a three-minute 120 pulse jog. In fact, it's downright dangerous.

Walking. As we said several chapters ago, this has been defined as the best exercise and for many individuals it may be the exercise of choice. However, it is hard to get the pulse to 120 by just walking. At the very least, you must walk briskly—"brisk" being defined as walking as swiftly as you can without running. Don't dawdle. If walking is one of the exercises you choose, we recommend that you do it at least once a day for at least thirty minutes at a stretch. In one study done to show the effects of walking as exercise, eleven women were allowed to eat whatever they chose with varying periods of daily walking interposed. All these women were overweight, and all had had trouble losing weight by means of diet alone. A daily log was kept by all the women in the group relating to their exercise cycle (a good idea for you, also, as we said at the beginning). In this study, every woman achieved a substantial weight loss with an average for the week of twenty-two pounds for the group but—and this is important—no weight loss of any extent occurred until the period of walking exceeded thirty minutes daily. The study concluded that the critical factor in achieving weight loss *by walking alone* was the motivation of the individuals to continue the exercise even if no results were seen.

But now we come back to that question we referred to at the beginning of the book: Can you lose weight through exercise alone, all else remaining equal? Chances are you could, though how much and—more important—for how long would you keep it off are issues that are debatable. Exercising for thirty minutes a day, though it may not sound like much, becomes a severe stumbling block for most people in the course of their daily routines. At least that is what we have found over the period of thirteen years during which we have been seeing patients for weight control. Exercise is something everybody talks about but after a few halfhearted attempts generally gives up.

That needn't be your situation any longer. Because of the revolutionary manner in which your Nine-Day Wonder Diet is set up, exercising is limited. Three minutes, three times a day. You can't say that much time will keep you too busy. And once you are done, your Wonder Diet will continue the benefits you have so quickly processed into your body. You might even say that your Wonder Diet continues working out even after you have stopped.

We don't want to create a wrong impression, though. If you want to walk for thirty minutes a day, we don't want to stop you. There are a couple of things you can do to lessen the tedium. First, plan ahead. "Where am I going to walk to for thirty minutes?" one of our lady patients asked us. "Half an hour is a long time just to walk." We pointed out to her that her walk really only lasted fifteen minutes, since the second fifteen minutes would be spent returning home. On that basis she felt the walk was considerably shortened and has walked regularly since.

Since it is hard to maintain an interest in the same scene, it is a good idea if occasionally you walk to *somewhere*. Visit a friend (provided you won't be offered something to eat when you get there), walk to a shopping mall or just along a different road or street. Keep your interest alive and your exercise will stay alive. One warning: If you walk *to* a shopping mall, or *from* it, that may well be exercising. But walking *in* it, while browsing through stores or window-shopping, is not. The only way your pulse will get over 120 under those circumstances is from the prices.

We can't leave the subject without once more referring to the overweight person's best friend—his or her dog. A dog on a leash is the greatest excuse for walking we know. Especially if your dog isn't housebroken.

Exercise combinations. You don't have to stick to one particular exercise. You may want to combine walking and jogging. This will cut down the amount of time spent walking. Jog until you get comfortably tired—not until your legs are ready to fall off. If you get that tired you'll need to rest. Once you rest in the middle of exercising, you have defeated the idea of exercising. The pulse rate has to go up to 120 beats per minute and stay there for the appointed time. Switching from one form of exercising to another helps use up body calories and breaks up the monotony of doing one exercise over and over.

Now the only form of exercise that we are discussing, and the only kind that works in weight reduction—we want to stress that: the ONLY kind that works—is active exercise. That is, exercise you do yourself, not exercise that someone does *for* you. How can someone exercise *for* you? Easy. You may not think of it that way, but such passive exercise on your part as getting massaged, using reducing machines or wrapping yourself in special bandages will not take a pound off you. Included in this list is having a staple put in your ear. According to this regime, you exercise this area by rubbing it when you are hungry and the hunger will go away. The only weight you will lose on these plans is from your wallet.

Active exercise is not an easy way to lose weight by itself; it is an easy way to *help* lose weight when combined with an efficient dieting regime such as the Nine-Day Plan. The following table will give you an idea what you may expect to lose from ordinary activities over a three-minute period:

Standing at ease	**2-3** calories
Light exercise	**85** calories
Walking slowly	**115** calories
Walking moderately fast	**215** calories
Cycling	**180-300** calories
Swimming	**300-700** calories
Skating (quick)	**300-700** calories
Cycling against the wind	**600** calories
Climbing	**400-900** calories
Running	**800-1000** calories

And, we suppose, no discussion of exercise would be complete without at least a mention of sexual intercourse as an exercise to help with your weight loss. Unfortunately, caloric expenditure is not all that great; it falls pretty much in the category of light exercise. It has been calculated that approximately seventy calories are lost by each party and most of this is fairly rapidly replaced by the eating that many people do afterwards or before. However, as an adjunct to whatever other exercise you elect, it should not be overlooked.

THE MUST ITEMS FOR THIS DAY

1. You will continue drinking your water—eight 8-ounce glasses. If you weren't quite able to manage this yesterday, today is your chance to improve. Ideally you got them all down yesterday so today will be even easier. Remember to space them out: 2 in the morning at say, 8 and 10 A.M.; 2 in the forenoon, perhaps at 11 and 12; 2 in the afternoon at 1 and 3 P.M.; and two in the evening, maybe at 5 and 7 P.M. These are only suggestions; you can devise your own time schedule, as long as you drink the water in some sort of divided dosage. A suggestion: If you find that you are having to get up a lot during the night to urinate, we would suggest that you complete your water drinking before 5 P.M. even if it means crowding the glasses closer together. It's no fun to miss sleep and, especially on this Plan, we want you well rested.

2. Today you will eat three dried apricots (halves) divided through the day as follows: one at 10 A.M., one at 3 P.M. and one at 10 P.M. This will take the place of the prunes you ate yesterday at these times. Again, these are sources of potassium.

3. You will continue to drink your two ounces of tomato juice or one ounce of orange-grapefruit juice half an hour before meals as you did yesterday.

BASIC MENU: Day 2
Breakfast

To be eaten no later than 10 A.M. and concluded by 10:30. We know that you probably like to spend more time at Sunday breakfast than you usually do at any other weekly meal of this nature, but your CBO won't allow that while you are on the Nine-Day Plan. So eat slowly and enjoy... but don't dawdle. If you get up later than 10:30, skip breakfast altogether.

½ cup berries with ⅓ cup skim milk
1 egg: fried, hard-boiled or poached
1 egg: cooked any way that is different from the first. You'll be surprised to find how much fuller you will be just from the eggs cooked two different ways. It's a sort of optical illusion for your stomach—a good trick to keep in mind.
2 strips of bacon or *1 breakfast sausage* (strictly optional)
1 slice whole-wheat or rye toast with ½ teaspoon margarine or butter
coffee, tea

Lunch

Not to be eaten before 1 P.M. Finish before 1:30 P.M. Do *not* attempt to combine a late breakfast with an early lunch, or brunch. This will throw off the CBO we have calculated into the plan.

1 shrimp cocktail (4 to 8 medium-size shrimp with sauce)
1 cup tossed salad: lettuce, tomatoes, onion, parsley with 1 tablespoon diet dressing or homemade dressing (see Recipes)
1 slice rye toast with ½ teaspoon butter or margarine
coffee, tea or 8 oz. of nonsugared soda.

Dinner

This meal is to be eaten no later than 7 P.M., and no earlier than 6:30. There is no special time for you to be done eating it. Tomorrow you have to go back to work and there are two days of great change in store for you, as you will see, so take your time with this meal. Eat slowly. Perhaps you have Sunday evening company. For many people, Sunday dinner is an event. There's no reason for it not to be even now. We furnish you enough variety for the entire day, so that you will be able to pick and choose and no one will even know you are on a diet. That's the way it should be, especially at dinnertime.

1 oz. of alcohol—Scotch, rye, bourbon, or such—but no mixed drinks using sugared soda, or juices whether sweetened or unsweetened. OR: 6 oz. dry white wine. Your choice—or neither, of course.

2 lettuce wedges (about ½ head), 3 slices tomato with 2 tablespoons oil, vinegar, garlic, herbs, pepper.

8 oz. broiled codfish

½ cup baked potato

½ cup any green or yellow vegetable

½ cup fruit cocktail

coffee, tea

SPECIAL: ½ oz. brandy (strictly optional)

SUBSTITUTIONS: There are no substitutions for Sunday meals.

ALTERNATE TIMES OF EATING

1. If you skip breakfast, you may eat lunch at 11 A.M. and finish by 11:30. You may then have an early Sunday dinner (which is the custom of many people) at 3 or 4 P.M. In this case you may require a snack before bedtime; either a large apple or pear is allowed.

2. If you sleep late but are up between 10 and 10:30 and desire breakfast, you may have it provided you skip lunch because of an early dinner. If dinner is at the usual time and you are hungry for breakfast, be sure that you are finished with it by 11 A.M. You should then eat lunch no later than 2 P.M. in order to achieve the proper CBO with dinner.

3. If you are up early for church and desire breakfast because you are hungry, you may move lunch forward by half an hour. If you are going to Communion and cannot eat breakfast until later, then do as in #2.

84

4. If you manage to miss breakfast and lunch, you must stay with the times given for dinner—either early or late; that is, do not eat either an early dinner before 3 P.M., or a "regular" one before 6:30 P.M. In no instance can you add to the dinner menu anything you've "missed" in the way of food from the previous meals.

5. Alcohol times are variable. You may save your drink for after dinner if you desire. Contrary to what many people think, alcohol enters the bloodstream at the same rate whether the stomach is full or empty. It is one of two substances that go directly through the stomach wall into the bloodstream, by-passing the intestine. The other substance is water.

ALTERNATE MENUS

You may utilize these rather than the basic menu discussed above if you desire. All include the 1 oz. drink of alcohol OR the 6 oz. of white wine. They all DO NOT include the ½ oz. of brandy. Where applicable, this addition will be so stated. These alternate menus, like those of yesterday, are prepared to be used in their entirety. Breakfasts, lunches and dinners must go together as we have placed them. These alternates are also to be used in succeeding cycles, depending on how much weight you have to lose.

Alternate Menu #1: Broiled Flounder

Breakfast 1 orange
½ cup cottage cheese
1 egg, boiled or poached
coffee, tea, ½ cup skim milk

Lunch 1 cup salad: 1 stalk celery, lettuce, radishes, tomatoes
asparagus tips (six) on 1 slice whole-wheat toast
½ teaspoon margarine
coffee, tea, 8 oz. diet soda

Dinner 6 oz. broiled flounder
1 cup salad: escarole, green pepper, tomato with "house
dressing" (see Recipes)
1 cup fresh berries (any kind)
coffee, tea

Alternate Menu #2: Shrimp en Brochette

Breakfast   ½ grapefruit
2 eggs, boiled or poached
1 slice whole-wheat bread
½ teaspoon margarine or butter
coffee, tea

Lunch   ½ cup cottage cheese
½ cup strawberries
½ cup orange sections
coffee, tea

Dinner   6 oz. shrimp
1 cherry tomato
2 cups salad: lettuce, tomato, cucumber, green pepper
½ cup rice
1 small ball ice milk (about the size of a plum)
½ oz. brandy

Alternate Menu #3: Crabmeat Cocktail

Breakfast   1 cup grapefruit slices
1 hard-boiled egg
1 slice whole-wheat toast
½ cup skim milk
coffee, tea

Lunch   1 small can tuna fish (oil drained)
3 lettuce leaves
2 oz. cottage cheese
1 apple

Dinner   4 oz. crabmeat cocktail
1 small baked potato
1 cup salad: onions, tomato, endive, radish
lemon juice
1 cup fruit cocktail (unsweetened grapefruit slices, orange slices, melon balls)
½ oz. brandy

Alternate Menu #4: Grilled Lobster Tails

Breakfast   ½ cup unsweetened grapefruit juice
½ slice whole-wheat toast

86

1 egg, fried
1 egg, poached or hard-boiled
1 cup skim milk
coffee, tea

Lunch ⅓ cup cottage cheese
⅓ cup radishes
½ cup cucumbers
½ cup raw mushrooms
3 lettuce leaves
house dressing
8 oz. diet soda, coffee or tea

Dinner 4 oz. lobster
3 slices tomato
½ cup green pepper
½ cup melted butter (unsalted)
1 cup cooked white rice
1 small ball ice milk
coffee, tea
½ oz. brandy (optional)
Snack: 1 apple or 1 banana

Alternate Menu #5: Broiled Fresh Mackerel

Breakfast ½ grapefruit
1 slice French toast (1 egg, 1 teaspoon oil or, preferably, use Teflon pan)
coffee, tea

Lunch 3 oz. shrimp cocktail
2 tablespoons cocktail sauce
2 oz. cottage cheese
1 cup mixed fruit: apple, orange, grapefruit, grapes
coffee, tea

Dinner 1 cup clam broth
3 oz. broiled fresh mackerel
1 medium-size boiled potato
3 slices tomato
3 lettuce leaves
house dressing

1 cup skim milk
coffee, tea
½ oz. brandy (optional)

Alternate Menu #6: Clam Casserole

Breakfast   ½ cup strawberries
4 oz. skimmed milk
1 cup oatmeal
coffee, tea

Lunch 3 oz. crabmeat or shrimp omelet (1 egg)
1 tablespoon oil
3 lettuce leaves
½ cup chopped onions
½ cup raw mushrooms
½ cup radish
house dressing
1 wedge melon
coffee, tea

Dinner   clams
1 cup rice
vinegar
spinach salad with House Dressing
1 small boiled potato
3 slices tomato
½ cup fruit compote
coffee, tea

Alternate Menu #7: Broiled Trout Almondine

Breakfast 1 orange
1 scrambled egg
1 slice toasted bread with ½ teaspoon margarine or butter
1 oz. Canadian bacon (about 1 piece)
coffee, tea

Lunch 2 oz. crabmeat cocktail
3 oz. cottage cheese
½ cup fruit salad
1 slice whole-wheat bread

½ teaspoon butter or margarine

coffee, tea or 8 oz. diet soda

Dinner 1 cup clam broth or any clear soup

3 oz. broiled lake trout

1 medium-size boiled potato or 1 cup rice

3 lettuce leaves

2 slices tomato

house dressing

coffee, tea

1 small ball ice milk

½ oz. brandy (optional)

Alternate Menu #8: Crabmeat Cakes

Breakfast 2 oz. orange juice

1 egg, fried

1 piece Canadian bacon

1 slice whole-wheat toast

½ teaspoon noncaloric jam or marmalade, or ½ teaspoon butter

1 cup skim milk

coffee, tea

Lunch mixed green salad: 3 lettuce leaves, 3 green pepper rings,
½ cup chopped onions, ½ cup raw chopped mush-
rooms, house dressing

1 slice whole-wheat bread with ½ teaspoon butter or
margarine

coffee, tea, 8 oz. diet soda

Dinner 1 cup mixed vegetable soup or clam chowder

4 oz. crabmeat cakes

1 cup rice

½ cup steamed broccoli or Swiss chard

3 slices tomato

special mayonnaise dressing or House Dressing

½ cup any berries

½ cup skim milk

coffee, tea

½ oz. brandy (optional)

Alternate Menu #9: Poached Salmon

Breakfast ½ canteloupe
2 oz. cottage cheese
1 slice whole-wheat bread
½ teaspoon butter or margarine
½ cup skim milk
coffee or tea

Lunch ½ cup coleslaw with vinegar dressing
4 oz. crabmeat salad: mushrooms, lettuce, onion, vinegar
    or lemon dressing
1 slice whole-wheat bread
½ teaspoon butter or low-calorie jam or marmalade
8 oz. diet soda or coffee or tea

Dinner 1 cup clear soup or 1 cup clam chowder
1 saltine cracker
poached salmon
1 small boiled potato
3 oz. steamed or wok-fried broccoli
1 cup skim milk
1 cup Jello
coffee, tea

RECIPES FOR SUNDAY, DAY 2

1. Broiled Flounder

You should use the whole, flat fish. Preheat broiler, lightly dust fish with flour, then brush with oil and place in broiler. Fish will broil in about 5-7 minutes. Serve medium; do not overcook. Baste during broiling with lemon juice, wine (dry), or vinegar. Drain fish and place on paper towel before serving to clear all grease.

2. Shrimp En Brochette

Have shrimp shelled and deveined. On skewer thread:
1 cherry tomato
alternating pieces of bay leaf
shrimp
raw mushroom
green pepper.

90

Repeat this process on as many skewers as necessary. Broil on grill, keep turning skewers during the grilling. Baste with Wesson oil. It may be advisable to parboil the peppers for five minutes before using.

3. Crabmeat Cocktail
Prepare canned or fresh crabmeat similar to shrimp cocktail on bed of lettuce. You may use shrimp-cocktail sauce. Place a raw radish in the center. One or two saltine crackers may be substituted for the ½ oz. of brandy.

4. Grilled Lobster Tails
Marinate 4 lobster tails for two hours in a mix of ¼ cup lemon juice, ¼ cup Wesson oil, 1 teaspoon paprika and 1 teaspoon Lawry's Seasoned Pepper. Add to taste, if necessary, ½ teaspoon Ehler's Garlic Salt. You may add ¼ cup mixed shallots, 1 drop Worcestershire Sauce.

Split underside of tails with scissors and break top of shell to straighten the tail. Brush a small amount of oil over the shell. Broil for five to ten minutes a side. Continue to baste with the marinade during the broiling process. You may garnish with asparagus spears—three per your own serving, no more. The dish serves 4, a tail for each. Good for outside grilling.

5. Broiled Fresh Mackerel

2 lbs. fresh mackerel fillets	2 teaspoons chopped parsley
¼ cup melted butter	1 lemon in wedges

Be sure you have fresh, not salt mackerel; salt mackerel has to be soaked in water for twelve hours and even then it will put weight on you from the salt. Dry fillets with paper towel, brush with melted butter and place in broiler, skin side up. Broiling takes about ten minutes until skin begins to bubble or turn brown. Baste with lemon juice during the broiling process. Turn only once and broil meat side. Sprinkle with chopped parsley and lemon juice. Use Lawry's Seasoned Pepper for taste. Serves 5.

6. Clam Casserole

2 dozen large clams
½ cup Wesson oil
½ cup lemon juice or
½ cup dry white wine
1 teaspoon chopped parsley
2 cups mushrooms

1 cup chopped onions
1 garlic clove or
1 teaspoon Ehler's Garlic Powder
½ bay leaf

Place clams in pan and cover with water. Bring to a boil, then reduce heat to a simmer, add ingredients above and let simmer tightly closed for one to two hours. You may thicken with tomato paste. Serves 6-8.

7. Broiled Trout Almondine

The gray sea trout has fewer calories than either the spotted variety or the lake trout; however, if you are at a restaurant you may take the lake trout if that is all they have. At home, the gray sea trout would be the fish of choice in this group. The broiling process is similar to that with the mackerel except that broken almonds are added while the fish is under the broiler. Sliced almonds may be purchased for this purpose but you can break up your own out of the shells. As in the case of mackerel or any other broiled fish, you may eat the skin.

8. Crabmeat Cakes

3 tablespoons margarine
1 clove garlic or 1 teaspoon
Ehler's Garlic Powder
ground pepper
¾ cup dry bread crumbs
4 tablespoons flour
1 cup skimmed milk

¾ teaspoon Lawry's Seasoned
Pepper
½ teaspoon Worcestershire
Sauce
6 oz. can crabmeat
1 egg, beaten
1 hard-boiled egg

Melt butter in pan with slices of garlic clove or powder stirred in. Remove garlic pieces once butter is melted. Blend in flour and skim milk until sauce boils and thickens. Add other condiments, then remove from heat. Divide sauce in half; to one half add the bread crumbs (¼ cup) and crabmeat. Mix, cover and place in refrigerator. When chilled, shape into small patties, dip in remaining bread crumbs and egg. Pan fry until brown, then serve with rest of the sauce, reheated with chopped hard-boiled egg and thinned with milk. Serves (about) 5.

9. Poached Salmon

We like to use salmon steaks here, but you can poach salmon fillets as readily. You may poach in a white wine if you desire; in that case discard the saltine cracker in this menu. The flavor of the fish may best be retained by adding a pinch of salt to plain water and poaching in this liquid.

MORE VARIETY DIETS AND HINTS FOR THE FIRST WEEKEND

Let's say you've less than ten pounds to lose. Your CBO can be accomplished more readily than in heavier individuals. This is true even if you've lost weight on another diet plan and found you just can't shake those last few pounds. We've treated a great many people on the Nine-Day Plan with just this problem. "I always get to a certain point and never can lose any more," one lady told us. "And I know if I don't get rid of the rest of this weight I'm going to put it all back on. And I've been depriving myself of everything for so long."

One cycle on the Wonder Diet was enough to bring this woman down to normal. You can do as well, even adding some variety foods to the standard diets in the preceding chapters. We can give you these because of the unique nature of the Nine-Day Plan. Remember, if you've more than nine pounds to lose, you can't use these variations quite yet—but take our word for it, the time will come.

TRY THE FOLLOWING SAUCE RECIPES

We've gotten a very enthusiastic response from our patients with anywhere from between three to ten pounds to lose by adding some of these sauces. Remember, their use is strictly limited to those of you with only nine pounds or less to go. Those with more to lose inhibit their CBO and don't get the proper benefit from the Nine-Day Cycle if they add sauces to their diet.

Tomato Sauce

1 No. 2 can of tomatoes	1 teaspoon Ehler's Garlic Powder
4 tablespoons safflower oil	1 bay leaf
1 onion chopped fine	1 can Heinz tomato soup

Put the onion and garlic in a saucepan and sauté in oil for from six to seven minutes. Add tomatoes, bay leaf, ½ can of Heinz tomato soup and cook till thick. Stir regularly. Add condiments, simmer to proper consistency. Add more tomato soup to taste. This sauce goes well with meat loaf, hamburger annd most fish.

Sauce Blanc

2 tablespoons safflower oil 1 cup skim milk
2 tablespoons flour Lawry's Seasoned Pepper

While oil is heating add flour. Stir milk in slowly, keeping heat low, then bring to boil and add seasoning. You may change the flavor by adding celery powder, onion juice, lemon juice, Worcestershire sauce. Does well with fish, and is great for vegetables.

Curry Sauce

4 tablespoons safflower or Wesson oil ½ cup chopped onion
2½ tablespoons flour 1 chopped apple
1 cup skim milk 1 cup of any broth
1 tablespoon lemon juice ½-2 teaspoons curry powder

Sauté onion in oil; add curry powder and apples. Blend in flour until smooth. Add broth, milk, bring to a boil. Add condiments. This is very good over rice and poultry.

A Cheese Dip You Won't Drown In

½ lb. cottage cheese 2 teaspoons dry onion soup
¼ cup fat-free buttermilk ¼ cup skim milk

Mix cottage cheese and buttermilk until well blended. Add onions and mix all in a blender. Add paprika and Worcestershire sauce to taste. DON'T dip potato chips... but this is good for raw vegetables such as celery stalks, carrots, radishes, and such. We never said you couldn't make a dip for your company that you, too, could enjoy.

IF YOU'VE TWENTY POUNDS OR LESS TO LOSE...

You may have been hovering at this weight despite trying diet after diet, regardless of how much weight you lost to get to this point. Or you may be just starting to go from here down to your proper weight. In either case it is perfectly all right for you to add the following recipes to your standard Nine-Day Diet if you desire. Again, we'd like to repeat that we are treating individuals with individual tastes and preferences, so we've taken the trouble to calculate the CBO at a number of different levels of overweight so as to present you with as many food preparations as you could possibly want—and that without compromising your weight loss.

Veal Scallopine

1 lb. veal slices
¾ cup flour
½ cup Marsala wine
2 tablespoons Wesson oil (or other vegetable fat)

lemon juice
1 clove pressed garlic
2 tablespoons chopped parsley
Lawry's Seasoned Pepper

Veal must be rolled thin. Sprinkle with flour and place in hot oil to brown. Add wine and allow to simmer. Sprinkle with pepper. When removing from pan and before serving, sprinkle with lemon juice and parsley.

Baked Veal In Milk

veal slices
1 egg
flour

¼ cup margarine
1 cup skim milk
1 cup water

Meat must be dry. Cut into pieces for serving, dip in egg and flour. Brown meat in hot margarine. Add milk and water mixture to casserole containing meat. Cover and bake for two hours. You may also use evaporated milk here.

Veal Chop Suey

¼ cup Crisco (or other vegetable fat)
2 cups diced celery
Lawry's Seasoned Pepper
1½ cups boiling water
2 tablespoons cornstarch paste

veal cut in strips
1 cup sliced onions
1 tablespoon molasses
2 tablespoons chop suey sauce
3 cups rice

Place veal in hot fat. Add onion, celery, boiling water, Lawry's Pepper. Simmer for forty-five minutes. Add sauce and cornstarch until thick. Serve with rice.

Brisket and Vegetables

2½ lbs. lean brisket
4 medium potatoes, peeled
3 stalks celery
2 small turnips
1 can Heinz tomato soup
2 teaspoons Lawry's Seasoned
  Pepper

1 large carrot, scraped
1 onion, sliced
string beans
1 teaspoon chopped parsley
paprika
Wesson oil

Heat oil in large pot, just a small amount to cover the bottom. Brown meat well on all sides, then remove and cut into slices. Add tomato soup and ¼ cup water and return slices of meat to pot. Allow to simmer. Cut up vegetables. Add condiments to pot, then add vegetables. Stir well. Table wine may be added to thin mixture if desired. Serve covered with parsley.

Spicy Cheeseburgers

1½ lbs. ground beef
¼ cup skim milk
½ lb. American cheese or Swiss
  cheese
3 tablespoons pickle relish

2 tablespoons mustard or
  horseradish
½ teaspoon Lawry's Seasoned
  Pepper
⅓ cup margarine

Blend into the beef the Lawry's Pepper and a sprinkle of black pepper/paprika. Press into patties; cover each patty with a piece of cheese. Mix pickle relish, mustard or horseradish. You may add ⅓ cup chili sauce or a few drops of Worcestershire sauce to this. Fry the meat patties on both sides, then remove to oven and top with dressing and cheese. Broil until cheese melts. No buns are necessary; one or two of these should fill you up fine.

Beans and Beef

1 tablespoon margarine
1 lb. ground beef
1 teaspoon Lawry's Seasoned
  Pepper

1 can Heinz tomato soup
1 can red kidney beans
½ cup flour

Heat skillet, add margarine, then add ground beef and stir until brown. Do not overcook. Add tomato soup and drained beans. Thicken with flour as necessary or thin with water. Pepper to taste. In our families we call this "slumgullion."

96

Shrimp Cantonese

1½ lbs. raw shrimp	margarine
½ teaspoon ginger powder	½ teaspoon cornstarch
2 scallions, chopped	1 cup chicken bouillon
Lawry's Seasoned Pepper	black pepper
1 egg, beaten	2 teaspoons soy sauce
garlic powder	

Mix cornstarch and soy sauce in ¼ cup water. Add margarine, pepper, ginger, garlic and the shrimps to a pan and sauté. Stir well. Add bouillon. Cook to boiling; let simmer for five to ten minutes. Now add starch-soy sauce mixture and stir until juice thickens. Add beaten egg, stir once and serve immediately. This goes well with boiled rice.

Oven-Baked Scallops

1 lb. scallops	2 teaspoons water
Lawry's Seasoned Pepper	black pepper
whites of 2 eggs	1 cup bread crumbs
2 teaspoons margarine	

Season scallops with both peppers. Beat together egg whites and water. Dip scallops in this mixture, then in crumbs, then in hot margarine. Bake in shallow dish for fifteen minutes at 450 degrees.

Stuffed Lobster Tails

4 lobster tails	1 teaspoon parsley
1 chopped onion	½ cup bread crumbs
garlic powder	2 teaspoons Wesson oil

Cut open bottom of lobster shell, and broil tails with cut surface to heat for five to ten minutes. Then turn over, cover with stuffing of onion, garlic, parsley, bread crumbs and oil. Broil for ten more minutes.

AND FOR EVERYONE:

House Dressing

However much you have to lose, you may incorporate the following into your first weekend's diet. We have referred to a "house dressing" in the previous chapter's recipes. Here's how to make it:

1 cup Wesson oil	1 teaspoon ground saccharine
¼ cup lemon juice	1 teaspoon salt substitute

Place all the above into a jar, cover and shake vigorously. Place in refrigerator, shake again before use. You may vary the flavor by adding ½ teaspoon paprika, dry mustard, or ½ teaspoon garlic salt.

Variations on the House Dressing

For more variations of the above (especially for those of you who are used to a diet being a "punishment" that puts you on peculiar and terrible-tasting meals) we offer the following:

1. Add to your house dressing (basic formula) ⅔ cup ketchup per cup of dressing and 1 teaspoon onion, well chopped or grated.

2. To a cup of basic house dressing add 1 teaspoon of any dried herb or 1 tablespoon fresh herb. See your local health food store. (Suggestions: tarragon, dill, oregano, basil, and so on.)

3. Add to your house dressing 1 tablespoon per cup of any low-caloric dressing. This will give you a delicious taste with even fewer calories diluted through the dressing than you'd get using the low-caloric dressing by itself.

4. For poultry you may even make a stuffing from your house dressing by adding 1¼ cups chopped oysters and bread crumbs to proper consistency. We will discuss this further on the "poultry days."

MAKE YOUR OWN MAYONNAISE

Yes, you can have mayonnaise. Many foods call for it and you can answer the call by making your own. That way you know just what ingredients you are getting and, by following our directions, you won't be disturbing your CBO.

1 egg yolk	black pepper
1 teaspoon dry mustard	1 cup Wesson oil
juice of 1 lemon	Cayenne pepper
¼ teaspoon Lawry's Seasoned Pepper	¼ teaspoon saccharine

Mix everything except the oil together. Add oil drop by drop until mixture thickens, then add oil more quickly. Mix in lemon juice. Refrigerate. Serve chilled.

Mayonnaise Variations

1. Instead of egg yolk. Use this variation if your cholesterol is above normal or in the high-normal range.

1 cup Wesson oil	1 teaspoon Lawry's Seasoned
4 tablespoons milk protein	Pepper
1 teaspoon salt substitute	½ teaspoon dry mustard
1 cup hot water	2 teaspoons vinegar
½ teaspoon black pepper	

Mix in a blender the vegetable oil and milk protein; add mustard, salt, peppers. Combine the water, lemon juic3 and vinegar and add to mix in blender at low speed. Turn blender up to high speed for less than a minute and mix everything together. Serve chilled. Incidentally, never attempt to store mayonnaise by freezing it. This can be dangerous. Make just enough each time for a single use.

2. Tartar Sauce

To your mayonnaise (1 cup) add 1 tablespoon chopped onion (grated works as well), 2 tablespoons chopped dill pickle, 2 table-spoons chopped parsley, 1 tablespoon chopped stuffed olives. Mix well. Use sparingly if you've more then ten pounds to lose because of the salt in the pickles.

3. Thousand Island Dressing

To 1 cup of your mayonnaise add a tablespoon of grated onion and 3 tablespoons chili sauce. Blend well.

4. Extra-Low-Caloric Dressings

Combine ½ cup of concentrated lemon juice with 1 cup of water. Add half a teaspoon of saccharine and ¼ teaspoon of any salt substitute. This dressing is good with salads or vegetables.

For tomato or cucumber combinations mix equal parts of lemon juice and soy sauce (1 oz.) with ½ teaspoon of saccharine and 1 teaspoon finely chopped candied ginger or ginger powder.

TAKE PAINS WITH FOOD PREPARATION

It should be obvious to you, now, that you should neither be eating to live nor living to eat, but eating *and* living and enjoying both. Food is important to you; take pains when you prepare it. A good deal of the reason you got fat was the overwhelming *availability* of food: it's quite possible to open a can, a box, a jar, a bottle, a tin...and eat without any preparation at all. The Nine-Day Plan does not allow for this; it forces you to become acquainted with what you eat by having either to have your food specially prepared by whoever does the cooking in your family, or having to prepare it yourself. Our suggestion is that while you are on the Wonder Diet you acquaint yourself with the actual cooking mechanisms by which your food is prepared. Help out in the kitchen; it's really the only way to get on a first-name basis with your lifelong enemy-angel: food.

As you can see from the recipes for this first weekend, you can prepare your food in many ways: by broiling, frying, barbecuing, baking. Eat it raw, if you like; steak tartare is not specifically indicated but it is a form of meat loaf. Use raw onions. Add a raw egg, if you like. Even if this particular dish isn't for you, you still have a lot of options open. You are restricted from regular deep-fat frying or breading, though we have allowed for a bit of each in certain recipes. It is important that you do not at any time during the Wonder Diet allow your palate to become bored. Try to prevent this from happening. One way to prevent boredom is to go out to eat. The act of changing your eating location may make a difference in what you eat and may be considered as part of your food preparation. However, we do feel that this should apply only to those of you who have nine pounds or less to lose. If you've more than this amount of weight to get rid of during your Nine-Day Cycle, you'd be better off following the precepts laid down in the first chapter, especially the suggestion that you eat in the same room for all your meals.

If you do go out, don't go all out. For some people, leaving home means disregarding their diet. When you go out, take us with you. We'll be watching you if you just keep us in mind. We promise we won't spoil your appetite, but we won't let you spoil your promise to yourself to get thin. That's reasonable, isn't it?

SEASONINGS
On your Nine-Day Wonder Diet you are encouraged to use a

great variety of seasonings. Employ them in moderation; don't make them the food. Some seasonings are salty and you must beware of them. Learn to read labels. Anything that contains sodium chloride, sodium citrate, sodium nitrate—sodium *anything*—should be used sparingly, if at all. Some seasonings you can employ fairly liberally: pepper, garlic, marjoram, thyme, rosemary, bay leaf, dill and cloves, for example. The following seasonings may be used only with caution: ketchup, cocktail sauces, mustard, horseradish, barbecue sauce. Most of these are dangerous not because of their calorie content, but because of their aiding and abetting role in water retention. If you are the cook for your family, salt the food very lightly and let each person add his or her own salt at the table. This is especially applicable to anyone on our Nine-Day Plan, but it is also a good habit for everyone to get into regardless of weight.

Some people count onions and mushrooms as seasonings, and so we will include them here. You may have slices of onion and ½ cup of mushrooms as free additions to any salads where they appear on your plan. Please keep in mind, though, that we are speaking only of raw onions and mushrooms, not the cooked variety. Cooking, depending on the method, will add calories to them and can disrupt your CBO.

NOW, ON TO MONDAY

Saturday was a meat day (beef, lamb or veal) and Sunday a fish or seafood day. Calorie Burn Out is activated by the dinner meal, with the rest of the day's intake of calories contributing to the total fat loss. You haven't taken more food than was allowed, though, of course, you may have taken considerably less. That's fine. Either way your body has been healthily, not excessively nourished and has already begun to prepare those extra pounds of longstanding fat for oblivion. In fact, if you haven't already lost weight, you will begin to lose very shortly just from what you have accomplished on this first weekend alone.

Tomorrow is Monday, a workday for most of us whether it be keeping a job or keeping house, and it is a workday as well for your Nine-Day Plan. You will be surprised to find what an easy workday it will be and how much extra energy you will have from your diet plan to bring to your other activities. Make sure you go to bed early enough tonight to get your full eight hours of sleep. You may well feel that your dream of being at your ideal weight is closer to coming true than ever before.

Chances are, it is.

6

MONDAY: THE FIRST FAST DAY

Let's be honest with each other.

We're going to assure you that what we're going to ask you to do on Day Three and Day Four won't make you die, get a headache, feel weak or dizzy, upset your stomach, interfere with your arthritis or make you tired.

In fact, it might have just the opposite effect.

You are going to assure us that you haven't already made up your mind that these things are bound to happen.

For Monday and Tuesday are going to be fast days.

We can hear you now. "You mean I can't eat anything? I've got to *starve* myself?"

Well, hardly. At the same time, what we are going to ask you to do has a definite, positive effect on your CBO, will help you shed weight quickly, will increase your energy level, make you function more effectively mentally as well as physically—and is so easy that after the first several hours you won't even remember that you are on a fast. There's even one more benefit: not having to bother with taking time to eat will give you time to accomplish a number of those chores that somehow you've never been able to get to in the course of a "normal" day.

FASTING, NOT STARVING

Therapeutic fasting—that is, fasting for some medical purpose—is not new. Every decade or so it gets "rediscovered" and a whole lot of noise is made about its efficacy in everything from losing weight to purifying one's soul. We're going to be practical rather than mystical, though, about our fast. On the Nine-Day Plan it is only an adjunct to help your CBO shed your unwanted weight. Remember, we said an adjunct. The Nine-Day Wonder Diet doesn't work by fasting alone. Fasting, however, is one factor among a specially selected and tested group of factors that give the Plan its rapid, easy-weight-loss character.

The word "fast" means a total or partial abstinence from food over a specific time for any one of a number of reasons. We use it to help promote and restore your body equilibrium. Fasts, however, are not uncommon in many religions as "penance days," just as "feast days" are celebratory. Occasionally, one reads of a "purification fast"—as in the case of the foodless vigil kept by a warrior before he could become a knight. We don't want you to think of your fast as a penance, but similarly, as a purification ritual. And fasting by no means should be thought of as "starving." In fact, no one could starve on the few fast days of the Nine-Day Plan. Even where a fast may be extended for months to lose excess weight, the individual on the fast does not starve—and we are not interested in your fasting that long. On this rapid Nine-Day Wonder Diet your weight loss is speeded up by the other factors that make up the Plan. If you do accept the fast days as a therapy, as a way to allow the internal environment of your body to reach a balance—homeostasis is the word the great physiologist Claude Bernard used—then you will indulge in them with understanding and pride in the accomplishment.

The fast days are not meant to be a punishment. Few of us enjoy being punished and if you cannot consider a total fast as anything but that, you will have to consider some of the alternatives to total fasting that you will find in this chapter. Some of our patients have told us that they regarded the fast days as a sort of "confessional." They used them to "make up" for their previous excesses with food. They'd "been bad" and now were being "disciplined" for it.

There's nothing wrong with thinking this way, provided you realize that fasting doesn't put things right for a future orgy with calories. But if you feel it necessary to take a stern guiding hand with yourself, you can certainly consider the fast days from that point of view.

It is this necessity to be overly stern with themselves or, on the contrary, to feel sorry for themselves and exploit the emotion of the moment, that makes overweight people call fasting "starving." Starvation begins to occur when your body has used up all available stored calories in the fat deposits and begins to break down its own proteins, the building blocks of the body. Take a look: Are your fat deposits empty? Are all your bulges gone, the clothes sagging on your frame? If so, you shouldn't be reading this book, let alone fasting to lose weight. But we doubt that is the case with you. True, if we were going to ask you to go on a long fast for weeks, or even months, we would tell you that *this* could be dangerous and that you should not do it without medical supervision. But for the two-day fast on this Nine-Day Plan, unless you have some already existing medical problem that would make fasting inadvisable, rather than getting *into* trouble with it, you'll get *out* of a lot. And we've never found that any of our patients needed medical supervision during the time of the fast. Most of them felt livelier and less in need of their doctor at this time than ever before. However, just for the sake of completeness, it may be a good idea to tell your family doctor that you are going on a two-day fast. Chances are, he'll be all for it.

HOW FASTING EATS UP FAT

It's easy to fast, and fasting has no age limits, especially for the time allotted on the Nine-Day Wonder Diet. We've treated senior citizens and young children; even infants may be placed on short fasts. Most of the difficulty with fasting—and some people consider missing one meal a fast of long duration—is the emotional sense of deprivation and its consequences. "I couldn't possibly fast for two days," one lady told us in horror. "Why, I could die if I miss one meal."

Chances are, if you weigh as much as she did, that you'll die

105

sooner if you don't start missing them all—at least for a time. Remember, your body is always eating whether you put food into your mouth or not. Your body is eating your fat... converting it into liver sugar and from there transporting it into the blood to be burned for energy, part of which is used to convert more fat into liver sugar. And so it goes, a never-ending cycle. The problem is that if you are overweight, you are putting food in much more rapidly than your body can utilize it. This is all right up to a point, but the more overweight you get, the more food you are storing. The body uses only a certain amount for its energy requirements, and less as you get older. So the breakfast you ate last week... well, you haven't eaten it yet; it's still there in your body waiting to be utilized. The fact that you've eaten it from the standpoint of putting it into your body *physically* only means that you've changed its shape from bacon and eggs, toast and coffee to an equivalent amount of fat. Before your body gets to eat *it,* it has to eat the breakfast from the day before as well as that day's lunch and dinner. And those from the day before that. And so, backward, in a long line of uneaten meals.

The idea of fasting is to give your body a chance to catch up. When this technique is combined, as in the Nine-Day Plan, with certain foods that help increase the speed of the body in utilizing its vast stockpile of calories, the number of actual fast days can be cut down.

We've said that it is easy to fast, and it is. Hunger may not even appear during the first day, and if it does we have some things for you to do that will modify it or even prevent its occurring at all if you don't want to take any chances. By the second day, your hunger probably will have gone—unless you break your fast with carbohydrate foods. (More on this later.)

The most difficult thing, many patients have told us, is to socialize while on the fast days. "Just too many temptations around," as one man put it. Well, we don't advocate withdrawing from society for these two days, but if you find that's what works best for you, it is only for two days, after all, and you might find some spiritual rejuvenation as well in the solitary confines of your own thoughts and hopes.

106

SOME PROBLEMS YOU MAY RUN INTO

Gas. One of the reasons we put you on the fast after a weekend of specific foods is to alleviate the problem of intestinal gas. Remember those snacks we said you could have? Raw vegetables prior to a fast may help prevent gas during the fast. At the same time, if this occurs, don't be alarmed; some people find it a normal concomitant to fasting. Usually it goes away by the second day.

Nausea. Very rarely do we find this happening during the type of short fast we propose. It is not nearly so uncommon during long fasts, when just the sight or smell of food may provoke nausea. For some people, nausea is a danger signal that tells them that the fast is over—they must eat. Not so on our fast. On the one or two occasions we are familiar in which nausea occurred, the individual had eaten or drunk copiously the day before starting the fast and was paying for it now. This, again, is why on the Nine-Day Wonder Diet, you are not plunged headlong into fasting but rather guided into it following a nutritive and food-selective period. NEVER start the Nine-Day Plan with a fast. We will have more to say about this in a later chapter.

Constipation. People tend to misuse this word almost as much as they do the word "hemorrhage." To the anxious eye, any sort of bleeding can be considered a hemorrhage, and to the tardy bowel a day's delay might constitute constipation. Keep in mind when you are fasting that since nothing is going in, very little may come out. Again, it is not abnormal to skip a bowel movement, or even two, on the fasting part of this plan. If you are one of those people troubled with constipation, the fasting days might contribute to it. To avoid a problem, we would advise you to clean out your lower bowel with an enema Sunday night before starting the fast days. This will prevent the material that is already there from becoming hard and more difficult to pass when the fast is over. Knowing that you will not be running into trouble with your bowels because of the fast days will also ease your mind.

Fatigue. Once again, we have never found instances of fatigue due to any portion of the Nine-Day Plan alone. But to make doubly sure, we do advise that you get enough rest. This applies to all the nine days you are on the Plan, but especially to the fasting portion.

107

We have said before that eight hours of sleep is a requisite. The problem is, most of our patients begin to acquire such a feeling of well-being from the Plan, including the fast days, that they tend to overdo normal activities. We must therefore caution you against this or a certain amount of normal tiredness, rather than fatigue, will catch up with you. It is also necessary—not only for the purpose of avoiding fatigue but also for maintaining good health—to take your multivitamin daily, as we have said in the beginning of this book. If you take your vitamins and get your rest, fatigue will not bother you. In fact, as we've noted, you'll feel more sprightly than ever in your life.

Exercise. There is no reason why you can't exercise during your fast days unless there are medical reasons for you not to do so. We have included exercise suggestions in this and the next chapter for the specific days. One exercise that you can always do, if you are in any sort of reasonable health, is walking. Both of us have fasted for much longer periods than this diet calls for and we have walked for exercise and thoroughly enjoyed it; in fact, we never felt healthier in our lives. So you can certainly do it for the two days on the plan.

Work. You should go to work. There is no reason why you need feel it necessary to take a "sick" day when these two fast days will probably be the most "well" days you've had in a long time. However, don't do work on the fast days that you wouldn't ordinarily do on days when you are not fasting. You're not trying to prove you're Superman or Wonder Woman just because you're on a Wonder Diet. The fact that you can fly in an airplane doesn't mean you can jump off the roof with impunity. At work, as at every other activity, do your normal job. As we keep saying, you're going to find it hard to hold yourself back, but remember that your body still has to strike a balance with your new energy. Give it a chance.

Feeling cold. It is not unusual for some people on this fast to feel cold. Usually it is the hands that seem to be affected, and almost always the problem is an exaggeration of one that already has existed for some time before the individual went on the diet. We have seen it only in women, but that doesn't mean it can't happen to men as well. Should you feel cold all over (it usually happens only at odd intervals, for greater or lesser amounts of time but usually for no more than a couple of minutes), drink the beverages we have supplied with the fast. If only your hands get cold (or colder than usual), this will dissipate of itself. More than likely, it won't happen at all.

Feeling warm. As with feeling cold, we know of no instances in which this has happened to someone who had never experienced this phenomenon before the diet was attempted. Women in early menopause (the so-called change of life) seem to be more susceptible; the stimulus of the fast may provoke more "hot flashes" than usual. Again, the chances of this happening are remote, but if it only happens to you and to no one else, as far as you are concerned it is 100 percent disturbing and of course you'd like to be certain nothing outrageous is going on. It's not.

Tension. You ordinarily may be the kind of person who is "uptight." We suggest that tension is your worst enemy when dieting, and certainly this holds true for when you are fasting. The effects of anger, grief, and other pressures of all sorts will be added to your desire to lose weight and to what you will regard as the tedium of fasting. No matter how pleasant the diet may be, no matter how easily you are accomplishing the fast, the "losing-weight situation" will be your scapegoat for all other forms of frustration. No diet, no fast, can possibly stand up to this sort of pressure, which will be magnified by thoughts of all the things you are missing out on, no matter how temporarily. So if you are subject to tension, or even if you aren't, it is a good idea to follow the principles of relaxation we will lay down for you a bit later in these pages. It is important that you approach the fast in as easy-minded a manner as possible. Otherwise you will be setting up self-defeating handicaps along the way. Remember, you are not the first person to be attempting this Plan. Many others have preceded you. Their successes are not only your safeguards but your foreseeable future if you will relax and let it happen.

The people around you. Can you imagine trying to defuse a live bomb with everyone around you screaming directions and telling you that you are doing it wrong? That's just about the situation when you try to fast with members of your family telling you how awful you look and how liable you are to drop dead at any moment. Something is bound to explode; usually it is your diet, of which this fast is a part. It is one thing to attempt this Monday fast and find that you honestly cannot go through with it. We have alternatives for you in that case; you won't lose the same amount of weight as if you had fasted completely, but you will still be on the Plan and you will still lose. You will also maintain your faith in the Plan so that you might be able to maintain a complete fast for the next cycle. But it is something else entirely to let someone else make up your mind for you and, in effect, force you off the fast. That is the first step to giving up the Plan itself out of sheer disgust, thereby losing your best opportunity to become the man or woman you really want to be. No matter how well-meaning your friends and relatives, they will have no knowledge or understanding of the purposes of the fast, nor of the principles on which it is based. As we have pointed out, tension is the last thing you need when undergoing any part of the Nine-Day Plan. To do it in dread of consequences based on unreliable information from confused family members is hopeless.

The best way out of this situation is to go on the Nine-Day Plan in the environment of your immediate family only. Don't tell anyone else: not friends, not in-laws—nobody. Your immediate family should realize that you are serious, that this is a medically proven plan—including the fast—and that if they have any questions about what you are doing they can read the book. That is the best explanation and its own proof of success. Once you've gotten down to your ideal weight, then you can tell people how you did it. None of them can say, then, that it can't work, that "you'll die trying." Success is something no one can argue with.

EXTRA ADDED BENEFITS

We've heard the following over and over from patients:

"When I fast even for only two days, the lines in my face seem to go away."

"My skin takes on a better color and texture."

"Your Nine-Day Plan, including the fast, makes blotches and

blemishes on my body tend to disappear; it's almost like getting back to a fresher, earlier version of myself."

One woman wrote: "It's impossible to describe the change that came over me after following your Nine-Day Plan. Right after the fast days my eyes became brighter, didn't have that constant strain I'd been noticing. And my husband says my skin looks ten years younger."

And from another: "Your Nine-Day Plan is simply ingenious—I especially am intrigued with the 'mini-fast' in the middle of it. I call it that because I've fasted before, generally for much longer periods of time than you advise. What puzzles me is that I've gotten results from your fast that I never got from longer ones. I've lost weight faster—and easier—and I have a great feeling of well-being that I'm almost ashamed of, it was so easily come by. As for sex, not only do I do it better (so I'm told), but I enjoy it more and want it more. Hooray for you and the Nine-Day Wonder Diet."

These comments are only a sampling. You don't have to envy people like these; you can become one of them. The same process is open to you as to them. The fact that they succeeded means that your success is just around the corner, depending only on how badly you want it.

SEX AND FASTING

One question that always comes up is: "What about sex when I'm fasting?" We tell our patients in the office: "Your fast does not include sex. Take all of this ingredient that you want." If you are like most people on our plan, chances are you will want more. And why not? The Nine-Day Wonder Diet is a rejuvenating experience. By the time you are done with one cycle you will look younger, feel younger...act younger. At least that has been the consensus of opinion from our patients. This rejuvenation is cosmetic in many ways apart from sheer weight loss. You will not only look more streamlined due to having rid yourself of all those projecting bumps and bulges, but your skin will look healthier, your eyes will shine and the general glow of good health will provide a more youthful glimmer to your overall appearance. Losing weight alone enhances your attraction, but how you may *look* to the opposite sex is aided by how you will *feel* and how you will project this. Many of our patients have told us that the Nine-Day Plan, especially the fasting, started them on a new, vigorous sex life totally unknown to them when they were fat. The energy they had previously expended on their fat was—in many cases for the first time in their lives—directed into sexual channels.

"I never thought of myself as particularly sexually desirable," one man, a bachelor, told us. "But since getting to my ideal weight on your Plan, I feel like I'm Casanova. I'm not embarrassed any more to be seen in public; in fact I enjoy it. Especially when I'm with a good-looking woman. Who would have ever imagined it?"

Who? Certainly not this man, who was well over two hundred pounds (at least sixty pounds overweight) when he started on our Plan. Even we wouldn't have imagined it. But there you are.

FASTING GIVES YOUR BODY A REST

There's nothing unhealthy about fasting, especially for the amount of time required by the Nine-Day Wonder Diet. Haven't you ever gone on vacation, taken a rest from the cares and pressures of everyday life, "recharged your batteries," as you might have put it? Well, your body also needs a rest from time to time, a release from the pressure of the food that you are constantly pushing into it. Eating the food, putting it in your mouth and swallowing it is an easy process; for most of us, far too easy a one. But the food at this point is only in the body physically, not chemically. Digestion is the chemical process of absorbing the food into the body proper, and this is a very difficult process, one of the toughest the body does. It deserves a rest from this rough, everyday job—especially when such a rest benefits not only your body, but you as a total person. Think of it this way: You'll be able to eat more and better in the long run by allowing the mechanism that serves the digestive process a rest now and then. Medical documentation has proved that fasting is beneficial to the inside of your body. We have proved, with the Nine-Day Plan, that it is also beneficial to the outside of your body.

WHAT HAPPENS TO HUNGER?

Are you a breakfast eater? Chances are that you would answer "yes" to this question, because the majority of people do eat breakfast. We've all heard the phrase "Breakfast is the most important meal of the day."

Why?

What's so important about breakfast? What seems to be most important about it is that it keeps the breakfast food companies going. Other than that, its main importance to breakfast eaters is that it keeps *them* going until lunch. Or so they think. The fact is, it's eating breakfast that prepares and makes you hungry for lunch. You don't believe this? Forego breakfast one morning and you will find, to your astonishment, that you haven't got those familiar lunch hunger pangs. Why is this? The explanation seems to lie in the fact that, as long as you are eating, you put your body on guard not only for the present meal but for the next one. Your mouth, your palate, your stomach are in a stimulated condition and, having tasted food, will hold out only so long before making you uncomfortable enough to give them some more. What stimulates them is the previous meal. If you do away with the previous meal, to a great extent you do away with hunger. During a fast, of course, there is no previous meal, and so hunger gradually disappears—not completely, perhaps, but to a great extent. It usually reappears by the fourth day of the fast, but you will not be fasting that long. You will be back on the eating portion of the Nine-Day Plan by then.

You can see, then, that hunger should not be a problem on your fast days. However, if you are still concerned that you might be uncomfortable, that fasting might still provide difficulties, that you might not have the "willpower" to get through this period, there is still another factor you can take advantage of.

THE "TOTAL CONTENTMENT" PILL

No, this is not a "diet" pill. It contains nothing that will make you jumpy, tranquilized or in any way interfere with any of your body functions except hunger. Nor is it necessary that you take it at all, for it will not cause you to lose any weight. But it will enable you to get through your fast days more comfortably. You can get it in any ıgstore without a prescription. There are a number of different trade names for it: *Culdrin* is one; *Pretts* is another. The functioning portion of this pill is 100 mg. of carboxy-methylcellulose. What is that and what will it do to you? methylcellulose, as described in Chapter Three, is an inert substance found in many vegetables. Your body cannot absorb it; in fact, it forms a good portion of the bulk for your normal bowel movements. When taken in pill form, as directed, it helps control hunger. How? Methylcellulose swells when it is combined with water. If you take it in the doses recommended (two to four 100 mg. tablets three to four times a day), and with the amount of water (eight 8-ounce glasses per day), that you will be drinking, you will feel quite comfortably "full." We want to emphasize that although your stomach will be filled, no part of this "stuffing" will be absorbed into your body. The methylcellulose will pass on down into your small, then into your large intestine, where it will form a large portion of your stool and be excreted. We have been using methylcellulose in our office for many years to help control hunger. We have given it to persons of all ages, as well as to individuals taking all sorts of other medications. We have never found anyone to have a problem with it; nor have we ever found anyone who later, when thin, couldn't get along quite nicely without it. Certainly on those days of the Plan that call upon you not to eat anything, you might find that you need a crutch to lean on. This "total contentment" pill, taken as we have advised, can certainly help get you through your fast days, and so, indirectly, can help you lose weight through the action of your own increased CBO.

If you like, you can of course continue to take this pill throughout the Nine-Day Plan. We have used it as well with our Food Intake Plan, on which the people involved have a great deal of weight to lose. While we do not feel that it is necessary to take methylcellulose through the nine days of your Plan, certainly you will do yourself no harm if this is your desire. We would hope, however, that the food we offer on the eating days of the Plan would be more than enough to content you. However, we do recognize that individual variation is such that an additional aid just might be necessary to turn the trick; don't be embarrassed if this is the case for you. Combining methylcellulose with the Nine-Day Plan is certainly in order if it

114

helps diminish an otherwise ravenous hunger. Chances are (and we have found this true in our office) that you'll only need it for one cycle of the Nine-Day Plan in any event, limiting it thereafter to the fast days. But this is your personal choice.

THE "MUST" ITEMS FOR THIS DAY

1. Liquids. You may drink all the tea, coffee, clear broth, lemon or orangeade that you wish. Make the lemon or orangeade with the juice of one fruit per one quart of water. Add artificial sweetening to taste.

2. Alternate between hot and cold liquids. This is important for it will help control your hunger and make you feel, psychologically, that you've had a meal.

3. Eight to ten glasses of water is a must, regardless of what other liquids you are drinking.

4. You may drink diet soda if you wish, but this must be limited to no more than two 16-ounce cans per day. We recommend the nondyed variety.

5. Be sure to take your multivitamin-mineral tablet on the fast days. If you wish you may take two of these, one in the morning and one in the evening.

6. If you have decided to take the "total contentment" tablet of methylcellulose during your fast, be sure to drink the requisite amount of water with each pill. The more water you drink, the better these pills will work.

Morning

When you get up we advise having a good cup of strong coffee or tea, preferably black, with artificial sweetener if necessary. If you must have milk, one or two teaspoons of skim milk will slow down your CBO somewhat, but it is better than sacrificing your morning beverage. Follow this drink with a full glass of water in about half an hour and continue alternating water with tea or coffee until noon. At this point, if you wish, you may have some clear consommé or bouillon, or you may want nothing at all. Remember to take your "total contentment" pill regularly, according to directions, if you have decided to utilize this aid.

Afternoon

You are probably still involved in your activities of the day and, aside from "missing lunch," have not thought too much about food. You may be quite proud that, in fact, this day is going so well and so swiftly despite the fact that you have basically eaten nothing. Whatever you do, don't get on the scale at this point in the flush of your enthusiasm. Many of our patients have done just this and found that they had either lost nothing, or had even gained a pound from the fluids they were drinking. At this point too much knowledge may be a dangerous thing, in that it could well discourage you from continuing along a path that certainly will prove profitable, if only you don't expect too much too soon. There is an axiom for chronic scale watchers: *The scale shows only how heavy you are, not how fat you are!* The weight you gain from fluids not only will come off, but it will take a lot of your extra weight with it. You will shortly be able to see this in inches lost and clothes that fit where once they tugged.

Keep in mind also that up to this point in the day you may have deviated from your normal routine very little. Many overweight people do not eat breakfast or lunch. We hear this from them all the time. The difference is that now you are missing breakfast and lunch as part of an overall plan, not out of the desperation of the moment—and maybe even after a binge, at that. Besides, the critical part of the day is yet to come.

Evening

Evening, for many people, overweight or not, begins with the four o'clock "snack." Now is the time when your hunger begins to creep close, and from now to bedtime you may find your good intentions being challenged. Now is the time your "total contentment" pill will make the most difference; now is the time your enthusiasm and willpower may come under attack. We have several suggestions to help get you through this period.

1. Take a "total contentment" tablet in chewable form. (You can purchase them for swallowing or for chewing.) Chew them when you feel real hunger in the background.

2. Drink black coffee. The caffeine in the coffee helps to control

116

hunger. However, if you can't drink coffee, even Sanka seems to help.

3. Keep yourself busy. The worst thing to do on a fast is to keep thinking about the food you are not eating. One of the reasons most people do their eating at night is that they've nothing else *to* do. If you've a hobby (and if you don't, get one), now's the time to indulge it.

4. If you are the cook for the family, and if you feel terribly burdened by preparing all the food for other mouths, take off from the job for two evenings. You'd be surprised how easy it is. After all, if you were sick in bed, your family would manage; they wouldn't expect you to drag yourself out of a sickbed to prepare dinner. And you *are* sick, sick from overweight. You'll be back preparing meals in forty-eight hours. Your family should be able to understand this, just as they should be able to understand why, whether you prepare the meals or not, you won't be eating them. It's strange how different relationships emerge from this part of the fast alone.

"I was terrified at the idea of not making dinner for the family," one of our women patients confided to us. "But when I told my husband and children about my fast, they were so pleased at my determination that it was wonderful. I think they actually enjoyed 'doing for themselves,' knowing they were really making it possible for me to stay on my diet." This same woman got to her ideal weight in two cycles on the Nine-Day Plan. Her husband made it a point to drop by the office to thank us for "giving back to me the woman I married." Yet, by his understanding and concern, he'd contributed enormously to her success.

5. Remember always that *you are eating.* Just because you aren't putting food in your mouth, that doesn't mean your body isn't having dinner. It is. It is busy eating one of those dinners you stored away last week. It is eating stored food from your fat. A goodly amount of your hunger is mental, not physical. Think it out instead of eating it up. You'll serve yourself better that way than by serving yourself more of what already ails you.

6. Look forward to weighing yourself when the fast is over. It is not unusual to lose four or five pounds over the two days; we've had patients who have dropped as much as ten pounds after the second day of fasting. We can't promise you that you will lose this much; we can promise that your loss will be diminished if you go off your fast.

7. Be sure to exercise, even if you only walk around the block for half an hour. It will get you out of the house and away from the food that everyone else is eating. When you have finished your exercise, have a nice, tall, cool glass of water.

8. Go to bed early. Take a book with you; read yourself to sleep. The sharpest part of your hunger will probably be over at this point, especially if you've taken your "total contentment" pills as directed. Going to sleep early will not only get you the proper amount of rest so necessary to the success of your diet; it will get you away from food and thoughts of eating. We've had patients swear to us they got fat from dreaming about food, but we've never been able to find medical evidence to this effect.

IF YOU CAN'T FAST ALL DAY

Don't feel ashamed of yourself if you can't maintain an all-day fast; there may be many reasons for this. And, don't forget, you may well succeed in this endeavor on your next cycle. However, rather than have you go off your fast on your own and lose the benefit of everything you've done so far on your Nine-Day Plan, we've allowed for such a possibility. This doesn't mean that we are negating what we've said so far about the benefits of a complete fast. However, there is room for everyone in this diet, and we realize that not everyone has equal stamina.

We mentioned just a moment ago that your loss will be diminished if you go off your fast. In order nevertheless to keep this loss as great as possible, even though it won't be as great as if you fasted all day, you can still lose substantially by following our partial-fast instructions. Please keep in mind that you are not obligated to eat everything on the list; the less you eat, the better. The items are here for your convenience.

PARTIAL FASTING: LIST #1
(DINNER ONLY)

For those of you who have made it through the day but are

118

showing definite signs of strain toward evening, you may eat the following, provided:

1. You are really hungry—uncomfortable in both mouth and stomach. (Don't mistake stomach "growling" for true hunger, and *don't* eat just because it happens to be that time of day.)

2. You must sit down and eat slowly. Chew well.

3. Don't wait until you are absolutely ravenous to eat something.

4. You can eat only a single item. Do not eat more of it than is allowed; you can *always* eat less.

Going off your fast today has nothing whatever to do with tomorrow. Tomorrow is also a fast day, and you will approach it as if you had not gone off today's fast. You must take this Plan one day at a time. There is no reason in the world for you to dismiss or in any way hesitate over tomorrow's fast no matter how you do in today's fast—whether you go off today for one meal, two or all three. That doesn't mean you've "failed." There are no failures on the Nine-Day Plan. There is only success—if you stay within the limits we've provided. Even if you falter on the fast days, you will still lose weight if you maintain the rest of the Plan. And remember, there's always another cycle coming to allow you to try once again. The only time you "fail" is if you go off the cycle altogether. Even here, you can pick up the next cycle and start over. You've every chance in the world to be a success.

To control real hunger before it controls you, eat the following. We have given you choices based on the number of calories you will be ingesting in each combination:

Choices for Dinner
(No earlier than 4 P.M., no later than 6 P.M.)
136-Calorie Total

1 cup clear consommé or bouillon (salt-free)
4 oz. chicken (breast only, no skin)
½ cup tomatoes, sliced.
coffee, tea.

(It is preferable to drink both coffee and tea black. If you can't, you may use Cremora or any other nondairy creamer that is similar. No

119

more than 1 teaspoon creamer per cup, and preferably less.) This ingredient may thus be added to the recipes below.

61-Calorie Total
½ medium canteloupe
1 piece Melba toast
coffee, tea

98-Calorie Total
¼ cup strawberries
1 hard-boiled egg
coffee, tea

127-Calorie Total
1 cup jellied consommé
2 oz. liver
½ cup cucumber
6 stalks asparagus
coffee, tea

123-Calorie Total
⅓ cup pot cheese
1 stalk celery
coffee, tea

110-Calorie Total
2 oz. serving plain yogurt
2 oz. shrimp, no sauce
coffee, tea

73-Calorie Total
2 oz. trout
½ cup cauliflower or
    mushrooms
lemon juice
coffee, tea

136-Calorie Total
1 orange
2 oz. crabmeat
1 piece Ry-Krisp
coffee, tea

135-Calorie Total
½ dozen clams
2 oz. mackerel
1 can diet soda

You may make up other combinations for yourself. You must not exceed 140 calories; in all instances eat the least that will satisfy your hunger. We would advise following the exact combinations we have laid out for you because we have calculated certain foods that will least interfere with CBO. If absolutely necessary, you may add calories up to but not exceeding 140 if the selection leaves room for this. If you have taken your "total contentment" pill the way we have advised, chances are that the selection with the least amount of calories will ease whatever hunger you feel. If you haven't taken the pills (and we want to stress again that this is not absolutely necessary, merely another convenience we have provided for your comfort) or you have taken them and still think you had better eat something, it would be worthwhile here to review the following points, which apply as well to breakfast and lunch this day, should you decide to make your fast as minimal as possible:

1. Make certain you are really hungry: empty in mouth and stomach, becoming acutely uncomfortable. Ask yourself: "Am I hungry, really hungry; would I eat something I really don't like?" If the answer to this is "Yes," chances are (and we are assuming you are being honest with yourself) that you are hungry. Wait for a little while beyond this stage to see if your hunger increases or diminishes—do not wait beyond the times allowed for dinner.

2. Time is important. You must not eat before or after the hours given.

3. If you have chosen one of our selections that leaves room for it, you may add calories to 140. *Do not do this unless it is absolutely necessary.* If you do add calories, try picking several items of low-caloric value rather than a single one that will provide the calories all at once.

4. Remember, you can always eat less than the number of items in any selection.

5. Do not combine items from one selection with those of another and, if adding calories, try not to repeat items that are on another selection. (Booklet-size calorie counters are readily obtainable; we have provided a partial listing in this book.)

6. Be wary of making *your* combinations at the very last moment. It is especially to avoid this that we have provided selections for you as well as given you foods that will least affect CBO. If you make up your own caloric list at the last moment you will likely be impatient and possibly careless. This is a corrosive combination when dieting; under such circumstances it is easy to add more than the allowed number of calories. If this should happen, you will adversely affect your CBO and that will cause you to lose much less weight.

7. Don't go to the opposite extreme and make up your dinner list way ahead of time. This can be defeating to the idea of staying on a complete fast. After all, you don't know if you are going to be hungry or not. If you say to yourself, "Oh, I'm always hungry for dinner," that's the best way to make hunger occur. Wait and see—just don't wait too long unless you are determined *not* to go

121

off your fast. If you can get through this initial phase of hunger, chances are that it will disappear, or at least diminish, as the evening wears on. If not, you always have our lists as a security blanket.

8. If you do add calories to our listings, or make up a menu of your own, stay somewhat under the 140-calorie mark rather than trying to get right on it or as close as possible. That way, if you make a small mistake in addition, or if you have added calories to those in the food by your preparation of it, you won't be going over the mark.

9. Again, we want to stress: *Eat as little as possible and, of course, no second helpings.*

PARTIAL FASTING: LIST #2 (LUNCH ONLY)

Your fast on this first day may only last to the afternoon. Don't be embarrassed if you find you really have to eat something then; don't feel that you have "blown it." We've provided for people such as yourself. Your weight loss will be slower than that of those individuals who can maintain more of a fast, but that doesn't mean it is any the less important to us. Certainly it shouldn't be any the less important to *you*.

One major point: If you find yourself hungry for lunch, don't assume that you will also be hungry for dinner. This may or may not happen. Let's not force any issues at this time, but rather handle each event as it occurs. Take one mealtime at a time. You may well find that your hunger will not recur for twenty-four hours—if at all. On the other hand, you may be unbearably hungry by each mealtime. We don't think this will happen, especially if you are taking your "total contentment" pill, but we will see. After all, the worst that can happen is that you will be unable to stay on the fast at all, and as you will see, we have provided for that as well. So don't worry. We have done all the worrying for you.

If you do eat lunch, you will lose less weight than if you fasted all day or even if you fasted until dinner. However, you will still lose if you stick to our guidelines. Our experience has clearly demonstrated that it is more efficient to your overall weight program to lose less weight over a longer period of time while maintaining your own *individual* well-being, than to try to copy someone else who is losing a lot on the same diet and be under a strain from trying to keep up with the other person's body chemistry. That sort of thing can only discourage you from the whole plan. One of the reasons the Nine-Day Wonder Diet has been so successful is that anyone can accommodate to it. Even if your first cycle is less than perfect, you will still lose a considerable amount of weight—weight that you have been unable to lose on any other plan. In addition, you are training yourself to make the next cycle even better. So your morale goes up while your weight goes down. That's important, isn't it?

Choices for Lunch
(No earlier than 12 noon, no later than 1:30 P.M.)

61-Calorie Total
½ grapefruit
coffee, tea (nondairy creamer
   included)

86-Calorie Total
1 medium apple
coffee, tea, diet soda

75-Calorie Total
¼ cup peaches (fresh)
¼ cup pears (fresh)
½ cup celery
1 lettuce leaf
seasonings to taste from zero-
   calorie list
1 can diet soda

50-Calorie Total
½ cup escarole
½ cup cabbage
½ cup green pepper
½ cup celery
coffee, tea (no cream), diet soda

98-Calorie Total
¼ cup cottage cheese
1 small lettuce leaf
coffee, tea

86-Calorie Total
½ cup eggplant
½ cup fresh or canned tomatoes
½ medium onion
seasonings to taste from zero-
   calorie list
coffee, tea

86-Calorie Total
½ cup celery
½ cup carrot sticks
½ cup tomato (fresh or canned)
1 lettuce leaf
seasoning to taste from zero-
   calorie list
coffee, tea, diet soda

90-Calorie Total
¼ cup grapefruit and orange
    sections (fresh or un-
    sweetened)
2 oz. yogurt
coffee, tea (black), diet soda

48-Calorie Total
6 asparagus stalks
1 piece Ry-Krisp or Melba Toast
coffee, tea

87-Calorie Total
½ cup endive
½ cup escarole
½ cup green pepper
seasoning to taste from zero-
    calorie list
1 tangerine
coffee, tea (black), diet soda

As with dinner, you may go with our lists or make up others for yourself. *The total number of calories must not exceed 100.* Try to do with less than that if you are able to take the edge off your hunger. Review here the checkpoints that we previously applied to eating dinner.

IF YOU REQUIRE LUNCH AND DINNER

We've said, earlier, that eating lunch is not a prerequisite to eating dinner; however, you may find, after thinking about it carefully, that you are hungry for both meals. We have found the following to be true:

1. Your chances of losing more weight are greater if you eat only lunch rather than only dinner.

2. If you eat both lunch and dinner you will not lose as much weight by the end of your cycle as if you had eaten only one of those meals. At the same time, it is not true that your weight loss will be inhibited twice as much if you eat both meals. The factor here varies greatly from one person to another. In some of our patients it didn't seem to make much of a difference whether they ate one meal or both. We have had patients lose between eight and twelve pounds on the Nine-Day Plan who ate lunch and dinner on both fast days according to our specifications. We certainly do not advise that you do this, however, if it is not absolutely necessary.

3. Those of our patients who did not keep the fast days in their entirety did not generally lose as much weight on the cycle as those who had. This is a comparison of only one cycle, though. It doesn't

124

mean that you still can't get down to your ideal weight on more than one cycle. In fact, you might be better off this way. We have had people get down to their ideal weight on three cycles, eating on the fast days. On the other hand, we've had individuals who did one cycle perfectly but never got to their ideal weight because, though they still had more weight to lose, they either went off their Cycle Balancing Diet or never completed another Nine-Day Cycle. Sometimes, therefore, you are better off being slow and steady rather than a star that quickly fades.

Should you require lunch and dinner, you may combine from the lists given a total not to exceed 100 calories for lunch and 140 calories for dinner. That makes a grand total of 240 calories beyond which you may not go. If you exceed this total you have seriously affected your Calorie Burn Out and the rest of the plan will have its weight-loss properties badly diminished. Again, we can't say you won't lose weight. You will, provided you adhere rigorously to the remainder of the plan. But you certainly won't lose as much as you should if you go over your 240 calorie total on *either* of the fast days. The more you go off any portion of your Nine-Day Cycle, the more of your thin chances you are fattening up, the easier it becomes to go off the Plan the next time. If you keep doing this, pretty soon you won't be on *our* plan at all—you'll be back on yours. And that's the one that got you fat to begin with.

When you combine your lists for lunch and dinner, try to pick those offering the least calories in either instance. Picking a 48 Calorie Total for lunch doesn't, of itself, leave you free to pick a 192 Calorie Total for dinner as a reward. Keep the count low so as not to count yourself out. At the same time, if you really and truly need to utilize all the calories allowed, they have been put there for your comfort and convenience...and your continued weight loss.

PARTIAL FASTING: LIST #3 (BREAKFAST ONLY)

You may be one of those people who wake up "hungry" and must have something for breakfast even if you don't eat the rest of the day. This partial-fasting list is mainly for you. It is *not* for you if you eat breakfast solely because it is breakfast time, or because you think breakfast is the most important meal of the day. The only people to whom breakfast is the most important meal of the day are the breakfast food manufacturers. You don't have to help "Quaker Puffs." You're doing enough puffing on your own just trying to get around.

Breakfast, for you as an overweight person, is the most dangerous meal of the day, and certainly on this fast day we strongly urge you to skip it. Remember what we said about one meal stimulating your mouth and palate for the next? That's what breakfast can do to you if you are not careful. At the same time, there are people who must have *something* to eat in the morning aside from coffee. If you are one of them, and if it would be a hardship to overlook this ritual, we can accommodate you and still have you lose weight.

Choices for Breakfast
(No earlier than 7 A.M., not later than 9 A.M.)

50-Calorie Total
½ grapefruit
coffee, tea (black)

40-Calorie Total
2 oz. plain yogurt
coffee, tea (black)

60-Calorie Total
2 oz. brook trout
coffee, tea

50-Calory Total
½ cup orange juice (fresh or
    canned)
coffee, tea (black only)

50-Calory Total
½ cup cranberries
1 slice Ry-Krisp
coffee, tea (¼ teaspoon non-
    dairy creamer)

60-Calorie Total
½ medium canteloupe
1 slice Melba Toast
coffee, tea (with less than 1
    teaspoon nondairy creamer)

25-Calorie Total
½ cup strawberries
coffee, tea (black)

50-Calory Total
½ cup fruit cocktail (fresh or
    water-packed)
coffee, tea (black)

126

THE TOTAL NUMBER OF CALORIES FOR BREAKFAST MUST NOT EXCEED SIXTY. However, unlike with lunch and dinner, you must adhere strictly to the list you choose for breakfast; you may add *no* additional calories to it. If you choose the 25- or 40-Calorie Total you cannot add thirty-five or ten more calories to bring the number up to the mark. We have done this to assure the success of the rest of the day for, while it is possible that you may eat lunch and not dinner, and quite likely you may eat dinner only, our experience has shown that most people who start off with breakfast will eat the other two meals as well. Again, that doesn't mean you *have* to. You may certainly eat breakfast, skip lunch, and not eat until dinner, or you may be that rare person who can have something in the morning and not eat again all day. The point is, *you can't be sure.* Who can tell at the beginning of the day what the end of it will be? And, as we have said, our experience, based on work with thousands of patients, indicates that most people will follow up breakfast, no matter how limited, with two other meals.

So if you take anything at all for breakfast other than coffee or tea, even if the calorie count is below sixty, you must count the meal contribution as sixty calories. There is no such thing as "carrying over" calories you did not eat at one meal to the next one.

COMBINING BREAKFAST WITH LUNCH AND DINNER ON A PARTIAL FAST

You may find that whatever you ate for breakfast is holding you pretty well. In that case you don't have to eat lunch; skip it. But if you feel that you need to eat lunch, regardless of how many calories you consume below the amount allowed, consider lunch a 100-calorie contribution. This means that having eaten breakfast and lunch, you have calculated so far an ingestion of 160 calories—with dinner yet to come.

There's no law that says that, having eaten breakfast and lunch, you *must* eat dinner; however, according to our statistics, that is usually what happens. And, again, no matter how many calories you take for dinner up to the limit, you must count it as taking the maximum allowed: a 140-calorie contribution. That makes your total for this "fast" day an assumed intake of 300 calories, or about one-twelfth of a pound.

At this point you may well raise your hand and cry, "Whoa. Hold on there. You mean I've gained weight? I thought I was supposed to lose weight on this plan."

Well, of course you are going to lose weight. In fact, you probably already have. We've played a bit of an optical illusion on you just to make a point. The explanation is simple enough.

First, you probably have not eaten all the calories we've insisted you calculate for each meal you've sat down to, so this weight gain of $1/12$ of a pound is more apparent than actual. But even if you have actually consumed all the calories to which you are entitled if you are hungry, the $1/12$ of a pound that you have theoretically gained will disappear in the poundage that you will have lost. It's like betting a nickel to win fifty dollars. Do you worry about the nickel, or are you more involved with the opportunity it has bought you to win even more?

True, had you done a complete fast today, you wouldn't have put on *any* weight and would probably have lost more than you did by eating. But this may have been something you were unwilling to try to cope with. That's all right. We've made allowances for you, given you a way to fast without really fasting, rather than saying to you: "Do it our way or not at all." That wouldn't help you very much, only rob you of the precious chance to go on a Plan that can make you thin. We want you to have every opportunity to lose weight; every chance to succeed. So we've calculated this Plan allowing for as many individual differences as possible. Take advantage of them, if necessary. You are, after all, an individual.

There is one other factor. The total number of calories you may take in, eating every meal according to directions today, is 300. It has been calculated that a total daily caloric intake of 300-360 calories is enough to provide for maintenance of the body's "lean muscle mass," but not enough to keep the body from burning its own fat supplies to get the energy it needs to keep itself at a normal working level. Of course, we're not talking about an everyday input of this amount. But even on a "fasting" day, if you have to eat and do so according to instructions, you can get by comfortably, without injuring your health, yet still lose weight. And that's crucial.

So follow the instructions we are providing and allow this revolutionary method of weight loss we have developed to work for you. Chances are that you will get results better than you ever hoped for—and you won't be left feeling dragged out, run-down, all in. You will, in fact, be bubbling with energy, ready to live your new life as a new, thin person.

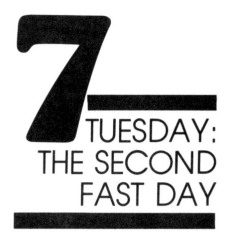

7
TUESDAY: THE SECOND FAST DAY

You may have noticed that we have done no preaching at you in this book. Well, we don't intend to do any. Nor do we feel it necessary to do a whole lot of theorizing about your weight, going into the reasons why you should lose and reviewing all the reasons why nothing you've tried has really worked well in the past. That's not our business. Our business isn't talking about your weight loss, it's showing you how to accomplish it; it's getting that weight off your back.

And that's your business too, isn't it? You don't want a rationale as much as you want results. Well, you're going to get results— lasting ones, so that once you have gotten to your ideal weight you can stay there, never get fat again, never have to promise yourself, "I'll start tomorrow." You've already started, and although you may not feel you've been dieting at all, you are now almost at the halfway point in your Nine-Day Plan. Easy, wasn't it? Well, the rest is just as easy... even easier, because the closer you get to the end, the more noticeable your weight loss becomes and the more determination you have to do the job well and get as many pounds off as possible.

130

YOU'RE DOING IT EASIER

You'll be surprised today to find that even in this short period of time, fasting has become a way of life. "I couldn't believe it" seems to be the general tenor of remarks made by our patients. "The second day of my fast I didn't have the urge to eat at all." One man says:

"I sat down at the breakfast table with my family, watched them put all the usual slop on their plates, watched them eat, swallow and even come back for more, without turning a hair. It was just as if I was removed from the scene. I wasn't hungry, sat there with my cup of coffee, and for one of the first times in my life felt *proud*. Do you know what kind of a feeling that is? I'd never missed breakfast before except on the first fast day, when I really had to hold myself back. Your diet has taught me more about myself than three psychiatrists—one of whom was a specialist in obesity control."

Even if you went off the fast yesterday, that doesn't mean you will of necessity *have* to eat today. Keep your mind unswayed. In fact, if you ate yesterday you may stand a better chance of *not* having to eat today because you know that the fasting portion of the Plan concludes today. You may not have been able to face the thought of not eating anything for *two* days, while not eating for one day is easily within your capabilities. Take it a third of a day at a time. And, if you did eat yesterday, remember, you didn't go off the track, you just took a bypass to reach the same point today as everyone else. With the amount of food you took in yesterday you can easily make it through today.

If you maintained a complete fast yesterday you, too, are in good shape to maintain a complete fast today. You've gotten into the swing of it, your hunger has diminished if not disappeared completely, you certainly don't want to lose the advantage you've gained by fasting—and in just a few hours your fast will be over and you'll be able to say to yourself: "I did it." Believe us, those are probably the three greatest words in the language. When was the last time you got to use them? Saying them to yourself is one of the true satisfactions in the world, one that very few people have a chance to indulge. Be one of the few. Finish the job you started, so that in a short space of time you can stand up and say to yourself: "I did it."

MORE ENERGY TODAY

Even if yesterday you felt a little tired and draggy, even if the headache you expected finally did materialize a little, you'll be astonished at the difference today.

"Totally washed" is how one of our patients, an airline pilot, described how he felt on the second day of fasting. "It was like coming back into the world with everything scrubbed, oiled and geared to full efficiency," a dentist told us. "Mystic, like being reborn" was a fashion model's comment. "And I lost five pounds just from the two days," she added.

Why this feeling of "total newness"? Some of it is probably just a "high" of self-satisfaction—completely warranted, we hasten to add. But there are physical benefits as well as psychological ones. A lot of the poisons in your bloodstream and tissues that have gradually mounted up as the byproducts of overeating can be removed by your body once it is given a chance to turn its energy to a total self-cleanup. It has to catch up with the work of sifting out the toxins that are already there, while continuing to attend to additional toxins that are being introduced in your daily meals. This process alone uses up a lot of energy—energy that is fueled by the process of burning up excess fat. The combination of this fat loss and the purification of tissues and blood from waste products that have been smothering your normal energy fires will certainly give you a feeling of coming back into the world with more zest, a feeling of complete rejuvenation.

It is a shame that so many of us live in a sort of limbo that we assume is "good health." It really is just so-so health, okay health—a compromise between feeling just fair and not feeling bad. The discrepancy between this health and the glowing radiance that comes from fasting *and* losing weight will be made abundantly clear to you today when, for the first time in a long time, you begin to feel vibrantly alive with energy and ambition to spare.

RELAXING TENSION

We spoke earlier about that uptight individual who brings all his problems to bear on his diet, just as previously he brought them to bear on his food. We told you then that we would have something to say about relaxing and, by this second day of your fast, it should be abundantly clear to you that this is an easygoing plan. We haven't given you anything really difficult to do, nothing that should make you nervous about your health; and we have not been inflexible as to the regulations for the basic plan. In fact, we've been most accommodating—as accommodating as we can be and still help you lose the amount of weight you should. That doesn't mean we can change your basically nervous character, if this is what you have. But you can change it; certainly you can modify it. While fasting you have the extra time to do something about this. It will help take your mind off food and it is a creative endeavor in itself, which you can put to use after your Nine-Day Cycle is completed, to help maintain your weight loss.

Here are some things to do that will help you to relax.

The breathing rhythm. This exercise in relaxing should be done at least three times a day. You can use the time you would ordinarily be spending at meals. First you must put yourself in a comfortable position. It doesn't matter if you sit, lie flat, or lie with your legs up. What is important is that you choose a position that takes as much strain off your muscles and internal organs as possible. You might want to put a cushion under your knees and another under your head. Let all your muscles go limp. Imagine your nerves going limp. Close your eyes.

Now start breathing. What's that you say? You never stopped? Well, we hope not; but you haven't been breathing the way we want you to. We want deep abdominal breathing right from the diaphragm, not the short thoracic pants that wind the air up inside you. Breathing abdominally means also that you are going to be breathing more slowly, not more than twelve times per minute, in long sweeping cycles. Breathe through your nose so that you don't dry your mouth out. Count as you breathe, visualize the air circulating inside you, through your lungs, right down into your abdomen. Let the dust settle; hold your breath as long as you can before exhaling. Count: One...two...three...four. On "one" you take the air into your lungs, as deep a breath as you can; on "two," instead of exhaling as you would in normal thoracic breathing, you let the air percolate down your spine, into your abdomen; imagine your whole body expanding as a bellows, feel each internal organ being brushed with life-giving oxygen. On "three" you start to exhale slowly, letting the air come out by itself, not forcing it. On "four" you gently constrict your abdominal muscles to drive the diaphragm upward and get rid of the "bad" air that is carrying with it much of the poisonous excretions of your body. The count is not an even one, the longest interval being from three to four as you allow the air slowly to escape. You should do this for at least fifteen minutes each time. Don't worry if you fall asleep. Try to keep your mind clear of unpleasant thoughts; concentrate on the one-two-three-four rhythm. If unpleasant thoughts intrude you will begin to feel the tension immediately; in this case get right back to counting and thinking about the air flowing restfully through your body like a wave flowing over sand. Remember that no one "accomplishes" relaxation. Relaxation is an absence of accomplishing; it's what happens when you turn off all interfering outside influences. Some people work so hard at "relaxing" that it only makes them more tense. Just concentrate on your breathing and the relaxation will come on its own. Incidentally, once you have the technique down pat you will want to utilize it all the time, not just on fast days. Don't do it right after eating anything, though; at that time your inner self is taken up mostly with digesting food and you won't be able to relax nearly as well.

The rag doll relax. The advantage of this method of relieving tension is that you don't have to sit or lie down. You can do it anywhere—providing you can get five or ten minutes alone. The first thing to do is to let out all the breath in your body in one long sigh of relief. Then let all your muscles go lax, your body go limp. Think of how a rag doll just sort of flops naturally upon any surface. As the air goes out of your body, imagine all your tension going with it. All that is left behind is your basic structure. Let your mouth sag open, your eyelids droop, your head hang. You can use a convenient wall for support if you like, but that isn't necessary. Even with your eyes partly open you can dissociate yourself from present surroundings, retreat from all external stimuli, concentrate totally upon doing nothing at all, upon an effortless floating. You will feel your arms and legs growing heavy; you may even sink to the floor.

If so, before you get up sit for a few moments; recondition yourself slowly to reality. You will feel fresh and able to face whatever may come. Just five or ten minutes of rag doll relaxing may give you more energy and soothing comfort than a whole night of sleep in which apprehensions flow just beneath the surface.

Be decisive. You've already seen how well this works; just making up your mind to lose weight, going on this Plan and sticking to it has already generated results you certainly would have never gotten if you were still just fiddling with the notion. Indecision is an energy waster, a leak in your valuable and not always quickly replaceable stamina fund. Feeling tired and worn even though you don't really "do" anything is a complaint we are constantly dealing with in our treatment of overweight people. The fact is, you *are* doing something to feel this way: mentally you are wasting energy, polluting your inner environment, poisoning the very wellspring of your existence. Indecision, procrastination and discontent may not drive you to drink but they will certainly drive you to food. And the energy you expend on them, while unfortunately burning up few calories physically, leaves you in poor condition to cope with the processes they lead to: worry, anxiety and apprehension about your weight. So the situation goes full circle; no wonder you find yourself weighed down with a feeling of fatigue. No wonder you are chronically tired. Add to this the daily physical activities you must perform plus the fact that you are carrying around a lot of extra weight while doing them, and the wonder of it is that you haven't simply collapsed under the burden.

Make up your mind, here and now, to cast the burden off. You *can* do it. No one *but* you can do it. Others have; others will. We've proved that in our office with the very diet you are now on. But indecision is a crafty foe; it sneaks up on you unawares, in the very midst of success, just when you think you've gotten the best of it. A little thing is enough to set it off—an extra bite of food, an extra drink, perhaps a party where you "forgot" your diet. Or maybe you weighed yourself and didn't lose the amount of weight you assumed you would to the extent you felt you were denying yourself. And suddenly, indecision is staring you in the face again. Is it all worth it? Should you go on? Maybe another diet would suit you better. Maybe it's just your "destiny" to be fat. Butterflies in your stomach along with too much food is a deadly combination. And, before you know it, there you are again, off your diet, eating away at everything you've accomplished, throwing away a thousand dollars because it isn't ten thousand dollars.

Once you've made your decision to lose weight on a specific plan, stick by it. Don't keep rehashing the idea, don't vacillate, hesitate or deviate. In fact, once you've made the decision, don't think about it at all. Just follow the path you've put your feet on to final success. You've chosen this diet plan wisely, based on all the evidence available to you. Give it a chance to work. The same holds true for anything you make up your mind to do. A clear-cut decision takes a load off your mind. Your Nine-Day Wonder Diet will take a load off your back as well. That, alone, should be a relaxing thought.

Be a little less than perfect. We've said it before and we'll repeat it now: you are only human. It's nice to have high standards, but you can't hold yourself so accountable for every little deviation from them that you get tense, nervous and finally give up a good thing because you've made it a bad thing. The old joke comes to mind of the people who couldn't bear reading about how bad cigarettes were for them—so they stopped reading.

Sure, you are going to do your best to stay on this diet. But you can't tear yourself apart over it. If you can't achieve success completely on the first cycle, achieve it partially. That's better than nothing. And try again next cycle. That's why we've set it up this way. We know that most fat people are defeatists. Rightly so, for most diets are defeating; they convince us that no matter how hard we try, we're fighting a losing battle. Not our Plan. We want to show you that no matter how little you try, you're fighting a winning battle. And when you try just a little harder, you'll win even more. So give yourself that chance—and that chance begins by admitting to yourself that you *can* do it... maybe not perfectly the first time, but *you can do it*. And the results you get will prove it to you.

Stop resenting. The middle-aged woman sat in our office crying. "I resent this," she said, wiping her eyes. "I resent being fat, having to come here, having to diet. I resent the way people look at me. I guess I really resent myself." Well, you may resent yourself. It's the easy way out of your problem. In effect, what you are saying is: I'm no good. I accept that. Therefore I may as well just give up the fight and eat.

We want you to know that resenting your situation is a process of self-poisoning that will eventually wreck your health. You can't resent what you are doing and follow any diet successfully. If you like, turn your resentment against us. Call us names, stamp on our book—get it out of your system through what the psychiatrists call "transference." Then pick up the book again and go right back on the Plan. It will be, suddenly, a lot easier to follow once you've taken your built-up resentment out on something. In this day and age too many of us hide our feelings, let the pressures build up inside, eat away at us. Then *we* start eating away, as one method of relieving them. Let the pressures out. Blow your cork. You'll feel a lot better for having gotten the poison out of your system.

Maintain a sense of humor. This isn't always easy in the face of adversity. The medieval poet François Villon comes to mind. On the occasion of his being sentenced to hang, he wrote: "My neck when stretched beneath the tree/Shall find how heavy buttocks be." True "gallows" humor. You can do the same. Stop taking yourself and everything else so seriously. That only contributes to your tension. We've always found that in talking to patients, as well as in writing books—whether about weight reduction or surgery—a sense of humor manages to keep everything in proportion. This is not to say that you should make a standing joke out of your being fat. That's only demeaning. But you can't treat it as the end of the world, either, and rock back and forth crying, "Nothing will help me." Nonsense. We'll help you; you're not so different from the thousands we've already helped. But every aspect of human experience, including death itself, has its wryly humorous aspect. Look at some of the inscriptions on gravestones: "Here lies John Smith. His wife finally knows where he's at." Maybe this doesn't sound funny to you, but perhaps for Mrs. Smith not taking death seriously was the only way to defeat it, to override a factor that most people consider pretty final. If human wit and ingenuity can keep death itself at arm's length—the better not to panic from its closeness—certainly you can do it with your weight. Stand away from it, look your problem up and down, consider some of its ridiculous aspects. We're not saying that you have to fall off your seat with laughter, but considering some of the things you've done to get that way and stay that way, you just may squeeze out a dry chuckle or two. And that's the first step toward taking yourself a little less seriously. It is also one of the most important weapons you will have for getting thin and staying thin. A good laugh is healthy. It not only releases tension and is soothing to your nerves and muscles, but it's a great exerciser for both muscles and bloodstream. In fact, it is one of the best (and least promoted) exercises there is.

Take up some sort of hobby. Of course if your hobby is eating, you'd better find something else to put your hand to, especially on a fast day like today. You may feel that taking up a hobby is easier said than done, but that's not really true. If you see it that way, you're just giving yourself another excuse to sit back and do nothing, get bored and eat. Incidentally, watching TV is not a hobby. Do something with your hands—whether it be woodworking, macramé, stained glass, silversmithing . . . the list is endless. You don't know how to do any of these things? It's easy to learn. The crafts explosion is everywhere; your local high school probably offers courses in many different crafts. Pick up the phone and call them. Join a class. If you are like the majority of our patients who have done this, you'll find it a lot more fun then eating. And you'll certainly know when you're hungry. That is when the sensation of emptiness in mouth and stomach overrides the interest in what you are doing with your hands. You'll be surprised at how seldom that will occur. Certainly having a hobby in which you take delight, feeling the thrill of accomplishment at seeing a work take shape under your guidance day to day, will help you take your fast days in stride, and will probably cut down on your intake during the eating days.

Don't be overcompetitive. In our practice we have many couples, and even mothers, fathers and children, who are dieting together. You might think this a good idea—as did we—for a mutual respect would be shared among the participants. In many instances this isn't true. A wife will say to us: ''You mean he lost more weight than me? And he wasn't even as faithful to the diet as I was? That really gets my goat." Or the husband will comment: "I think she's sneaking things into my meals that aren't on the Plan so she can lose weight faster than me." Even the children aren't spared in this frenzy of overstriving. A woman and her young daughter were on the Plan together. The woman lost more weight than the daughter. "You see," she crowed, "even though I'm older than you, I can still do things better." The daughter burst into tears.

When you overcompete—and most of this is done almost instinctively—you place not only yourself but those around you under a lot of tension. This will all reflect back on your eating pattern. It's nice to have a drive to succeed; we don't want you to lose that. But you don't have to run everyone else over on the way, end up feeling guilty... and fatter.

THE MUST ITEMS FOR THIS DAY

1. Liquids. You will continue to drink all the tea, coffee, clear broth, lemon or orangeade you want, as you did yesterday. Remember to alternate between hot and cold liquids. Do not doubt that you will feel fine. Drink all your liquids slowly; take small sips and let each linger in your mouth, making every one an experience in itself. That's what gourmets do. Be sure that when you are drinking you are sitting down. NEVER GULP. Think of what you are doing, why you are doing it and how close you are now to succeeding.

2. Continue with the eight to ten glasses of water.

3. Take the multivitamin-mineral tablet as before.

4. Take your "total contentment" pills as you did yesterday. If you did not take them yesterday, there's no reason why you can't start taking them today. However, if you did take them yesterday it isn't a good idea not to take them today as well. Your hunger, put off from yesterday with the pills, will hit you harder today without them. Of course, if you took no pills yesterday and wish none today, you don't have to take them. Your hunger, in this case, will be pretty well unnoticed today as compared with yesterday.

INSTRUCTIONS FOR THE DAY

You will do pretty much the same as yesterday. It might be well

139

here for you to review your reactions during yesterday's fasting activities. Even if you had some sort of discomfort then—whether a mild headache or some slight feeling of weakness—that doesn't mean you are bound to have the same reaction today. If you do, take whatever remedies you would ordinarily. Lie down for a while if you should feel weak. This will pass; it may just be due to a momentary drop in your blood sugar. Rest assured that your body will readily acquire more blood sugar by breaking down your fat. As for a headache, you are certainly at liberty to take a couple of aspirin. You might well have gotten the headache whether you were dieting or not; don't be so quick to blame things on your diet that you would have to accept as facts of life ordinarily.

One warning about aspirin, however. We suggest that if you are going to use this drug you take Bufferin or use coated aspirin (this has a couple of trade names; ask your druggist which he has in stock). This is so as to avoid even the remotest chance of getting an upset stomach from plain aspirin—which will tend to affect an empty stomach lining in this way much more readily than one that is protected by food. There are people who cannot take aspirin at all; whatever you do take should be no problem just because you are fasting. The point is, we don't want you suffering with a headache or any other bodily problem just because you are fasting. You aren't supposed to be a martyr. You've been enough of a martyr being fat.

We mentioned the possibility of constipation. If you ordinarily have difficulties with this, fasting will not help them. In fact, you may feel that the condition is exacerbated by the fast. The phrase "fast and loose" does not apply to you. At the same time, fasting is just as feasible for you as for anyone else. You may take milk of magnesia or any other laxative that is noncaloric. Be careful of those that are chocolate-coated. Read labels. We want you to be as comfortable as possible during your fast; we realize that life goes on and your body has other functions that must be attended to in addition to losing weight. The tendency of many diet plans is to disregard such functions, to subordinate everything to the dieting process. We realize that this is impractical, uncomfortable and unnecessary. At the same time, we want to re-emphasize that if you don't ordinarily have trouble with constipation you should not be disheartened if you find that your movements are irregular or even missing during the fast days. They will shortly get back to normal as the eating days recommence.

BREAKING THE FAST

Even though we are not talking about a fast of long duration, we have found it a good idea to give specific directions as to the best way to break the fast. Although it is usually only after many days of fasting that the body loses its immediate power to handle and assimilate food, we have had instances in which individuals experienced various types of discomfort by breaking their fast on whatever foods happened to be available. There is also the question of timing to consider. Our best success on this Plan has occurred with patients who waited until the morning of the next day to break their fast, rather than the evening of the fast day itself. If you break your fast on the evening of Day 4 rather than on the morning of Day 5, you may be saddling yourself with a sudden hunger that will possibly cause you to go off your diet. On the other hand, the advantage of breaking your fast in the evening is that the next morning you can, if you wish, start off immediately with the breakfast menu rather than waiting until the noon meal. A lot depends on how you have adapted psychologically to the idea of not eating for two days. It's really a matter of using your own good sense as a guide. If hunger has completely vanished, you might as well wait until morning to break your fast. In that case, even if breaking the fast does cause hunger to return, you will shortly be able to satisfy it with lunch. If you are already feeling somewhat hungry before you break your fast in the morning, you would probably be best to break it as close to lunch as possible, though not any closer than an hour and a half. We like to allow that much time for the fast-breaking to occur, so that your digestive tract will become reabsorptive to food and peristaltic action (intestinal motion) can stabilize.

We have selected your fast-breaking foods with the utmost care. Please do not use any items other than those that are allowed for this purpose. If you break your fast on the morning of the Day 5, you may consider this breakfast; if on the evening of Day 4, you may choose breakfast from the menus stated as such on Day 5.

141

FAST-BREAKING MENU
(USE NO OTHER FOODS)

1. Have half a glass of orange juice (preferably fresh and un-strained). Take at least five minutes to sip it. Sit down while doing this.

2. In thirty minutes take half a grapefruit or a medium slice of canteloupe.

3. In thirty minutes take half a glass of carrot or tomato juice,

In each of the instances given above, care should be taken to eat and drink the substances as slowly as possible. If you gulp them down you are quite likely to get a stomachache and ruin a lot of the advantage that you've gained from fasting by not being able to follow the plan of Day 5. If, on the other hand, you follow instructions, you will find breaking your fast a comfortable and pleasant activity, to be followed by further weight loss without having to fast anymore.

If for some reason you cannot take orange juice, you may substitute unsweetened grape or pineapple juice. But do not do this unless it is absolutely necessary as these ingredients may affect your CBO.

All items used to break your fast should be eaten at room temperature. This permits ease in digestion. Ice-cold and iced juices are to be strictly avoided at this time. Remember to SIP SLOWLY. This may sound silly, but one way we've gotten patients to make sure they are taking their juice in as slowly as possible is to chew it. Not only will this cause a slower ingestion, but the chewing motion will mix saliva with the juice and make the digestive action of the stomach easier. It will also tend to make you feel more full and allow more time before hunger comes.

We have used this method of fast-breaking with people suffering from all sorts of complaints, including chronic constipation and hemorrhoids. Excretion for such people can be just as much a concern as intake (if not even more so). Rest assured that if you follow instructions, this worry, too, will become a thing of the past.

IF YOU CAN'T FAST
ON THE SECOND DAY

This might be the case whether you've fasted on the first day or

142

not. Many factors may come into play, mainly emotional ones. Someone may have gotten sick in your family, you may have had to go out of town unexpectedly—while at first glance these may seem to have little bearing on whether you are fasting or not, many people will feel that such situations interfere with the rhythm of fasting and so will go off their fast. This, while not very efficient, is a very human reaction. So don't call yourself names and, again, don't think you've "failed." You may also stop fasting on the second day just because your hunger may get too much for you, you are bored with the fast or you have got yourself into a nervous state. (Review the section on "Relaxing Tension" at this point.) Whatever your reason for not being able to fast the second day, regardless of what you did on the first day, if you will follow the suggested lists for bending, rather than breaking, your fast, you can still lose a considerable amount of weight. *You must not substitute the Partial Fasting Lists of the first day for those of the second day.*

You may not combine any of the lists of the first day with those of the second day.

You may not add calories to any of the Partial Fasting lists of the second day. If you choose a menu with fewer than the day's allotted calories you must stick with it. This doesn't mean that you should automatically pick the menu offering the most calories. Remember, the less you eat, the more you will lose. At the same time, we want you to be comfortable.

Remember, you can always eat less than the amount shown but never more.

PARTIAL FASTING: LIST #1
(Dinner Only)

Once more we start with the meal furthest away, assuming that you can get this far if you really want to. If you got this far yesterday, you can certainly do so today; and if you didn't quite make it yesterday, it was still good practice for near-perfection today. Remember, if you get through the day to dinner, that should involve a minimum of discomfort; many people do this routinely. You needn't think of it as fasting at all, but rather as a rehearsal for the fasting that you will be more comfortable with next cycle (if such is necessary).

143

Choices for Dinner
(No earlier than 4 P.M., no later than 6 P.M.)

100-Calorie Total
1 cup clear bouillon, salt-free
4 oz. shrimp (no sauce)
coffee, tea (black)

50-Calorie Total
2 oz. brook trout
coffee, tea (black)

100-Calorie Total
½ cup strawberries
2 tomato slices
1 lettuce leaf
wine vinegar and seasoning
    from zero-calorie list
2 oz. lobster or ½ doz. clams
coffee, tea (black or ¼ teaspoon
    nondairy creamer)

100-Calorie Total
2 oz. canned salmon (no oil)
lemon juice
½ cup lettuce or endive
tea, coffee, (¼ teaspoon non-
    dairy creamer)

100-Calorie Total
½ cup lettuce
2 slices tomato
½ cup mushrooms
½ cup green peppers
wine vinegar or ½ teaspoon
    house dressing
4 oz. shrimp or scallops
coffee, tea

80-Calorie Total
1 cup jellied consommé
1 medium apple
coffee, tea (¼ teaspoon non-
    dairy creamer)

50-Calorie Total
2 oz. chicken breast (no skin)
coffee, tea (black)

75-Calorie Total
2-inch wedge honeydew melon
2 tomato slices
1 lettuce leaf
wine vinegar and zero-calorie
    seasoning
coffee, tea (¼ teaspoon non-
    dairy creamer)

80-Calorie Total
6 stalks fresh or canned as-
    paragus or ½ cup cauliflower
½ cup raw carrots
2 lettuce leaves
½ cup fresh or canned tomatoes
wine vinegar or lemon juice
ιcoffee, tea, (¼ teaspoon non-
    dairy creamer)

50-Calorie Total
1 cup clear salt-free bouillon
2 oz. shrimp or scallops
coffee, tea (black)

Do not make up for yourself combinations other than those shown. The total number of calories for dinner this day must not exceed 100. Your "total contentment" pill can help keep your calories below this amount. Review those portions of our last chapter that relate to the possibility of your eating dinner, keeping in mind that the lists for this second fast day are final.

SNACKING IN PLACE OF DINNER

Quite often we are asked the question: "Suppose I'm not hungry for dinner between the hours you allow, but I suddenly find I'm hungry later in the evening. Can I eat then?" Originally we said no to this request, but circumstances may allow a modification of this stance. If for some reason you are going to be going to bed later than usual this night, you may utilize *any single item* from the above lists as a snack—this provided it is done no less than two hours before you intend to go to bed. You may have unexpected guests, some family emergency, or just decide to do something that will keep you up considerably later than is your habit. In this case, we see no reason for you to be uncomfortable, and possibly snacking at something you shouldn't have at all. But don't use this as a built-in excuse to eat. The allowance doesn't apply unless you will be up a couple of hours past your "normal" bedtime. And, of course, the eight hours of sleep will still apply, so you will probably miss breakfast on the other end if you go to bed late enough to qualify for a snack. Incidentally, this proviso does not apply to yesterday's fast—only to today's.

PARTIAL FASTING: LIST #2
(Lunch Only)

You may have gotten by without lunch yesterday, only to find that you really would like something to eat at this time today. That's all right—provided you are really hungry and not just taking a break from work or keeping somebody company. You can take a break from work and read a book, or keep somebody a lot better company by not interrupting your conversation with food. But if you are beginning to get uncomfortable and don't wish to fight it further, or are afraid that the discomfort will grow beyond the time allotted for lunch, then you may select from the following. You may not add calories to these lists though, as usual, you may take fewer than are shown.

Choices for Lunch
(No earlier than 12 noon, no later than 1:30 P.M.)

50-Calorie Total
½ cup canteloupe balls
1 lettuce leaf
½ cup cucumber
coffee, tea (black), diet soda

37-Calorie Total
1 cup clear salt-free bouillon
1 piece Ry-Krisp
6 stalks fresh or canned asparagus
coffee, tea (black), diet soda

50-Calorie Total
½ cup cabbage
½ cup mushrooms
½ cup green peppers
½ cup cucumber
seasoning from zero-calorie list
coffee, tea (¼ teaspoon non-dairy creamer)

25-Calorie Total
1 cup clear soup without fat
½ medium pear
coffee, tea (black), diet soda

50-Calorie Total
1 lettuce leaf
½ cup green peppers
½ cup celery
½ cup mushrooms seasoning ₁ from zero-calorie list
coffee, tea (black), diet soda

25-Calorie Total
½ cup cranberries
coffee, tea (black)

50-Calorie Total
½ cup radishes
½ cup cucumber
½ cup escarole
½ cup raw cauliflower
wine vinegar or lemon juice
coffee, tea (½ teaspoon non-dairy creamer), diet soda

50-Calorie Total
1 cup salt-free consommé
½ small fresh grapefruit
coffee, tea (black), diet soda

The total number of calories must not exceed fifty. Try to do with even less than that; as you can see, it is possible to eat something and take in much less than the maximum number of calories allowed. Do not combine items from one list with those on another.

TODAY'S LUNCH-DINNER COMBINATION

As with yesterday, you may eat lunch and not want dinner, or you may. We have allowed for the possibility. The same factors apply as did in the previous chapter. Should you require lunch and dinner today, you may combine from the lists herein a total not to exceed 100 calories for dinner and 50 for lunch. That is a grand total of 150 calories—but they must be split the way we've shown. Again, you can't carry over unused calories from one meal to another.

PARTIAL FASTING: LIST #3
(Breakfast Only)

For your breakfast choices this day, assuming that you need to eat something in the morning, you must refer back to the lists of food for yesterday's breakfast. The total number of calories permitted for breakfast today is the same as that of yesterday: 60. That will give you a total for the day of 210 calories as the absolute maximum. DO NOT EXCEED IT. Unlike yesterday, you may not add calories to any of the lists to bring them up to the 60-calory mark. If you make a selection totaling fewer than 60 calories, stay with it. Nor should you make up your own lists. Be strict with yourself. Don't worry about not having enough to eat. There's a good eating day coming up. In the meantime give your body a chance to have a feast—on your fat.

COMBINING ALL MEALS TODAY

If you do eat all the meals today (naturally you don't *have* to and we would prefer you didn't), you will not lose as much weight as someone who maintained a complete fast. Nor would you expect to. If you also ate all meals yesterday, your weight loss will be somewhat further diminished. But this doesn't mean that you won't lose weight. In fact, if you do not deviate from the guidelines we've set, *you will still lose a considerable amount of weight*—weight that in all likelihood would have had more poundage added to it had you not been on the Nine-Day Plan. How much weight you will lose depends on how much weight you have to lose. We've had patients who have eaten all meals on both fast days, according to directions, and have still lost five pounds by Wednesday, Day 5.

That is still a pound a day—an excellent loss, with more to come on the rest of the Plan. And, by eating even less on the fast days next cycle, or by fasting completely one or both days, you can lose even more weight. So you don't have to worry about "all that willpower that is required to fast." We're showing you how to semi-fast, and next cycle it's quite possible that you will be ready to try complete fasting. If not, do just as you did on this present cycle. It may take you a little longer to get rid of those excess pounds (depending on how many there are) than someone who has fasted for both days of the cycle, but you needn't mind that. The Plan is still effective for you, as you are losing weight at the rate of speed that best suits you. Remember, the loss of just one pound makes you more of a person, less of a fat person. As a person you are entitled to the same opportunities to lose weight as everyone else. Our diet will provide you with this opportunity, modified slightly for your personal convenience.

AND IF YOU'VE FASTED

If you have fasted for both days of the cycle you are entitled to feel pretty good—mentally and physically. You've probably learned a good deal about yourself and have a good deal more confidence in attempting any situation.

Tomorrow is the first time in forty-eight hours that you will be eating. It is time to decide whether you want to break your fast tonight or wait until tomorrow. Review the way of breaking your fast that we discussed earlier. Whether you will do it tonight or sometime tomorrow morning is your choice. The longer you can carry your fast within these limits, the better. Remember, fasting is not eating anything for a specific period of time. That's the definition we'd like you to keep in mind. Many people have their own definitions. One of our patients told us: "My definition of fasting is a day I don't eat cake."

So, if you can wait until tomorrow and give yourself those extra hours, chances are you will lose more weight. But whatever time you break it, you will have learned a truism about fasting that you can pass along to your relatives and friends who ask you, "How was it?"

Your answer: "Nothing to it."

8
WEDNESDAY: THE FULL PROTEIN DAY

You are now truly beyond the halfway mark. We offer you congratulations—but you must admit it hasn't been so bad. In fact, you should be enjoying the change from your previous eating habits with all the guilt feelings you had to swallow along with the food. Chances are you've never done so well on any other plan; and you can't say it's been boring. You haven't had to interrupt either your daily work habits or your social obligations; certainly we hope you haven't. We don't want you to be "better" than we ask you to be. As one young lady said to us:

"Oh, I've been so good on your Plan. I just sat home and ate when and what you told me to and I lost a lot of weight... but I was so lonely. I told my boyfriend I didn't want to see him for the nine days because I felt he would tempt me off my diet, and I wouldn't see my folks because they'd tell me it wasn't good for me to eat like that, so all I did was sit home and read and watch TV. I cried a lot."

Please don't do this to yourself. Our Plan isn't meant to be a punishment. There are many diets that are meant to be just that, but not ours. Dieting is basically a lonely business; we want to make it less so, as well as more productive. You'll perform any activity better when you are having a good time, when you are *not* depressed. Remember we told you that the Nine-Day Wonder Diet is a *human* plan for human beings. Don't treat yourself as anything less just because your previous experience with diets has taught you that the "stricter" you are with yourself, the better the diet will work. The most extreme example of this came from a middle-aged man who was a partner in a large corporation. "I did better than you said," he told us as we calculated his weight loss. "I fasted for the entire nine days."

When we asked him why, he said: "I wanted to be strict with myself."

What he was really saying was that he wanted to punish himself for being fat. Since he couldn't do that on our Plan, he selected another. That's fine—but if you do this don't tell yourself you are on the Nine-Day Wonder Diet. You aren't. We don't want the credit—or more likely the complaints—that other diets can provide. That's why we devised this one. And on this one you *can* socialize, you *can* enjoy yourself, you *can* eat. There are variations to the Plan; you will find these in a later chapter. But we don't want you making up your own variations. Because if you do, you will be right back where you were before—on *your* plan, not ours. And yours is the one that got you fat.

Furthermore, if you, like the young lady in our first example, are a teenager, don't hide from your parents what you are doing because you think they'll tell you "it isn't good for you to eat like that." What really isn't good for you is the way you have been eating. Let your parents read this book. We've treated many hundreds of teenagers in our practice, and quite successfully. We've treated adolescents successfully where other types of treatment, other diet plans have failed. If, after reading this book, your parents still aren't convinced, we'd be happy to have them write to us, care of the publisher, with their questions. We'll get the message—and we'll reply. We did so with our previous book describing the Food Intake Plan, *You Can Be Fat-Free Forever,* and we'll do so with this one. Why should we take this kind of time? Because, as many of our patients tell us with some surprise: "You're really interested in my problem."

We are. *We're interested in your weight!* We're interested in your losing unwanted pounds as quickly and as healthfully as possible. We hope we don't want to see it happen more than you do, because that wouldn't help you. YOU want you thin—we're already there. We lost our weight many years ago by our own reduction methods. We never gained it back. You can do the same. All you have to do is follow our instructions. And, as we started this chapter out by saying, you are, today, more than halfway there, more than halfway down the road to proving to yourself that friends can look at you and say: "You look ten years younger; what have you been doing to yourself?"

GETTING ON THE SCALE

Yes, today you are going to weigh yourself. We certainly hope you've been staying away from the scale until now. Constant weighing can become a discouraging habit. Perhaps you've shared the experience of one of our patients:

"I went on this diet and nothing was said about not weighing myself. Well, I was on it twenty-five minutes and weighed myself seventeen times. Nothing happened, so I quit."

"Quit weighing yourself?"

"No. quit dieting."

Does this sound exaggerated? Well, it isn't. Not a bit. We've had it happen among our patients. Remember, curiosity killed not only the cat, it can do the same to your incentive. You will get results from your Nine-Day Plan if you stay with it, probably better results than you ever imagined you would achieve with any diet plan. But these results don't always show up right away regardless of how much effort you feel you are putting in. Give your body a chance to catch up with your determination. That's why we've kept you off the scale until today.

It might be a good idea for you to review here the discussion we had in the first chapter relating to weighing yourself. Keep the following things in mind:

1. Weighing must be done first thing in the morning, nude, immediately after urinating.

2. If you do not weigh yourself at this time, forget about weighing yourself at all.

3. After this morning's weighing, you will not weigh yourself again until we tell you to.

4. The above holds true regardless of how much weight you've lost or how much weight you think you should have lost.

5. Whatever your weight may be, remember that the diet is not over; there are several days still to come.

6. Most of your weight will be lost (as far as the scale is concerned) at the tail end of the Nine-Day Cycle. Of course, you may lose a lot before then, but don't be disappointed if you do not.

(In fact, we've had many patients lose a number of pounds on the tenth and eleventh days after the cycle has been completed, based on what they did on the previous days. So don't be surprised if this happens to you in addition to your losing an excellent amount of weight during the plan.)

7. If you find today, on weighing yourself, that you've already lost a lot of weight (and this may well be the case, especially if you've been observing a complete fast), don't get so carried away by your success that you disregard the part of the diet still to come. All this will do is turn your immediate success into something considerably less. That would be a shame, especially since you've such a heaven-sent opportunity to turn it into something so much more just by following the remainder of the plan.

8. You just may find that by this morning you've already lost all the weight you have to lose. You may have had only eight or seven pounds to lose...and they're gone. There you are, halfway through the cycle at normal weight. What do you do now? You MUST FOLLOW THE REST OF THE CYCLE. If you don't, you may gain back the weight you've just lost. In fact, you may gain more. The reason for this is not difficult to understand. You've lost most of your weight through not eating anything for two days. If you go off the Plan now, revert to the way you were eating before without giving your new weight loss a chance to "lock in," you will be right back in trouble and you will find it harder to lose the next time. The Nine-Day Plan is calculated not only to get you to lose but to get you to keep off the weight you have lost. It is therefore essential that you carry the cycle through to its conclusion. Failure to do this will be worse than if you hadn't gone on it at all; you'll gain everything back.

HOW YOU WILL EAT TODAY

You will be eating three good meals today. They will be composed mostly of protein. This doesn't mean there will be no fats or carbohydrates, but these items will be held to a minimum. Each meal on the basic Plan will start with half a grapefruit. There are two exceptions to this. If you are breaking your fast this morning, rather than last night, you will not eat the breakfast meal. You will substitute for it the fast-breaking foods from the previous chapter. Then you will carry on with lunch and dinner. If you cannot eat grapefruit, you may substitute half an orange, one medium pear or half a large apple.

Now, let us say something right here. Many of our patients insist that they can't eat certain foods, strictly out of habit. "I'm not a meat person," one woman said. "What I really go for is bread." *You* may not think you're a meat person. But that's all in your head. You *know* that you can change your outlook mentally if it will result in your changing it physically. Get all these fat notions about food out of your mind. We can't promise that you'll suddenly adore foods to which you've long been unaccustomed, but if these are the ones that will help you lose weight in a rapid, healthful manner, and are, in addition, prepared in a most palatable style, you may just find that you've been missing a lot *not* eating them. So stop categorizing yourself as a certain *kind* of eater. That's only how you've trained yourself to eat, probably out of circumstance. These circumstances can be changed, must be changed if they interfere with your goal of getting to your proper weight. If you go on the Nine-Day Wonder Diet and don't come out at the end of the cycle losing weight *and* inches from thighs, waist, chest and hips, then you have done something wrong; you haven't followed the Plan. "I followed the Plan pretty much," said the woman who wasn't a "meat person." Well, following the plan pretty much just isn't much—and you won't lose much either.

Today you must eat all meals to whatever extent you are able— no skipping, even if you only eat a small amount. There is one exception: breakfast. If you are breaking your fast today, do eat all the foods indicated for that meal. You must stay within the allotted time span for all meals; this, of course, is true whether you are following the Basic Menu or one of the alternatives. If you don't care for the Basic Menu you may use an alternate menu this time and try the Basic Menu next cycle, assuming that you have more weight to lose than one cycle can get rid of. We'll have more to say about this later on.

All meats should be medium-lean to medium-fat.

WHAT YOU WILL EAT TODAY

1. Eight glasses of water, divided through the day. We must keep stressing this factor. Because of the varying nature of the Wonder Diet from day to day, what we don't specify many people won't do. You may, as before, substitute club soda or seltzer for the water and you may add lemon juice to it if you want to give it flavor. You may also drink more than the eight glasses if you wish; though this will help with your hunger, it doesn't mean that you will lose weight faster, though you may. We are going to continue to be very specific about your activities with food through the remainder of the cycle, just as we have been so far.

2. You will eat three medium apricots today. You may have them canned provided they are water-packed, or you may have them fresh. DO NOT EAT THE DRIED, UNCOOKED ONES. Eat one apricot with each meal. This is a must.

3. Today you will drink half a cup (four ounces) of skim milk with your lunch and dinner ONLY. Sip it slowly; it will help fill you up. If you wish, you may use this item as a snack between lunch and dinner, and between dinner and bedtime. Do not take your skim milk less than two hours before retiring for the night.

4. Take your multivitamin-mineral tablet today with one of the glasses of water you will be drinking. It makes no difference what time of the day you take it.

5. You may or may not be using your "total contentment" pills today. We suggest that these might help make you more comfortable, but this is something you will have to decide for yourself. If you are planning to use them, use them throughout the day routinely, and remember to drink your water with them as necessary.

We have provided a Basic Menu as the ideal for the day; it contains the listed ingredients that the majority of our patients

154

found best for losing the maximum amount of weight for the day. However, alternate menus will follow; a minority of our patients found at least one of them more helpful than the Basic Menu. We suggest that you try the Basic Menu first; if that is not entirely comfortable for you, then try an alternate one next cycle. Remember, you are an individual and, as such, deserve individual attention and an allowance for your individual variance from the "norm." The Nine-Day Wonder Diet is unique in allowing for exactly this kind of variance. We are not trying to "cut you down to size." We *are* trying to find the best and most efficient routine for you to follow in getting to your ideal weight as rapidly as possible— thereby allowing your own body to cut *itself* down to size.

So look over the Basic Menu, and then study the alternatives. Choose the food routines that seem to "fit" you best. Chances are, these will be the ones that will do the most comfortable job for you. We have found many of our patients enthusiastic over this acknowledgment of their individuality. It gives them a sense of self-importance which, we hope, you will also find. That is one of the things that leads to successful dieting. Remember always, it isn't the diet that is important. *You* are important. You must choose the routine that you can best live with.

BASIC MENU: DAY 5

Breakfast ½ *grapefruit (or alternate fruit as previously noted)*
4 oz. ground beef (broiled only)
onion, scallion, parsley (seasoning amounts only)
pepper or salt substitute to taste
coffee, tea (½ teaspoon nondairy creamer)

Lunch ½ *grapefruit*
4 oz. steak, oven- or pan-broiled. Use Teflon pan; no butter or oil.
seasoning to taste from zero-calorie list
coffee, tea, diet soda (1 can only allowed today)

Dinner ½ *grapefruit*
4 oz. liver or veal or lamb (see Recipe section)
coffee, tea

For those of you who broke your fast last night and want to push your weight even more rapidly than the Basic Menu for today will do, you may use the following version. One caution: You *must* eat *everything* on this one without fail:

MORE RAPID LOSS
BASIC MENU: DAY 5

Breakfast ½ medium cantaloupe
4 oz. medium-fat beef, broiled or fried in Teflon pan
black coffee, tea

Lunch ½ grapefruit
4 oz. medium-fat beef, broiled or fried in Teflon pan
black coffee, tea

Dinner ½ medium cantaloupe
4 oz. medium-fat beef, broiled or fried in Teflon pan
black coffee, tea

On this more rapid variation of today's plan you will not take the skim milk or the apricots that are a part of the Basic Menu. You *will* take your multivitamin-mineral tablet and your "total content-ment" pill (if you're doing this anyway).

Remember, on both the Basic Menu and the More Rapid Loss Basic, you can eat less than is shown but you cannot skip an ingredient altogether. Eat what you can and don't worry about eating meat for breakfast. It is all right to take less than the amounts given, providing you take the time to sit down and decide. Even if you've convinced yourself that you aren't hungry, sit at the table. Your body has the right to make up its own mind.

Eat today at the following times only; if you miss these times you will have to miss the meal. You can't make it up at another time; you will be disturbing your CBO and you will not lose all the weight we have calculated you should lose for the cycle.

TODAY'S TIME ZONES

Breakfast: No earlier than 7 A.M., no later than 9 A.M.
Lunch: No earlier than 11 A.M.; no later than 12:30 P.M.
Dinner: No earlier than 6 P.M.; no later than 7:30 P.M.

If your work hours or school schedule conflict seriously with these times we have provided, you will have no recourse but to change the schedule of our times to suit your necessity. But always

156

remember to keep the time proportions the same as we have them. Don't change our schedule for convenience only. Don't change our schedule unless it is absolutely necessary. And never eat dinner later than 8 P.M.

We have found that when patients change our eating times, the diet never seems to work quite as well for them. One reason may be that any modification you make perhaps tends to give you a false feeling of control. This may lead you, unconsciously, to start changing other aspects of the Plan as well. Be very cautious about changing any part of the Plan. It works too well as it is for you to begin tinkering with it out of mere caprice.

ALTERNATE MENUS TO TODAY'S PLAN
Alternate Menu #1: Combining Beef and Veal
Breakfast *1 orange*
1 egg (poached or hard-boiled)
2 pieces Ry-Krisp
coffee, tea
Lunch *1 cup clear soup, salt-free*
4 oz. chopped meat
seasoning to taste from zero-calorie list
½ cup chopped onion
2 slices green pepper
coffee, tea
Dinner *4 oz. tomato juice*
6 oz. veal dish (see Recipe section)
½ cup chopped eggplant
½ cup cucumber
coffee, tea

Alternate Menu #2: Combining Beef and Veal
Breakfast *½ grapefruit*
2 oz. chopped meat
1 thin slice of bread
coffee, tea
Lunch *4 oz. steak, broiled*
salt substitute and pepper to taste; zero-calorie seasonings

2 slices tomato
4 oz. lettuce
coffee, tea

Dinner ½ cup tomato juice
4 oz. broiled veal chops
coffee, tea

Alternate Menu #3: Combining Beef and Lamb

Breakfast 4 oz. orange juice
2 oz. "breakfast steak"
1 piece thin whole-wheat toast
coffee, tea

Lunch ⅓ cup cottage cheese
½ cup grapefruit and orange sections
½ cup watercress
1 cup skimmed milk

Dinner 1 cup bouillon
4 oz. lamb dish (see Recipe section)
coffee, tea

Alternate Menu #4: Combining Beef and Lamb

Breakfast 1 orange
2 pieces Ry-Krisp
coffee, tea

Lunch 4 oz. bean soup (any kind so long as nothing else is added)
4 oz. rack of lamb
½ cup lettuce
½ cup cauliflower
coffee, tea

Dinner 4 oz. strawberries
4 oz. beef dish (see Recipe section)
coffee, tea

Alternate Menu #5: Combining Beef and Liver

Breakfast ½-inch wedge honeydew melon
⅓ cup cottage cheese
1 slice thin bread
coffee, tea

Lunch *8 oz. mushroom soup (not creamed)*
4 oz. liver dish (see Recipe section)
coffee, tea
Dinner *½ cup fruit cocktail, fresh or water-packed*
4 oz. roast beef
coffee, tea

Alternate Menu #6: Combining Beef and Liver

Breakfast *4 oz. pineapple, fresh or canned (water-packed)*
4 oz. hamburger, oven- or pan-broiled (Teflon)
1 piece thin bread
coffee, tea
Lunch *6 oz. portion of liver dish (see Recipe section)*
coffee, tea
Dinner *8 oz. onion or 4 oz. tomato soup*
⅓ cup cottage cheese
½ cup lettuce
½ cup celery
½ tomato
½ cup onion
½ cup raw mushrooms
seasoning to taste from zero-calorie list
coffee, tea

Alternate Menu #7: Combining Lamb and Veal

Breakfast *1 orange*
1 egg (poached or boiled)
2 pieces Melba toast
coffee, tea
Lunch *4 oz. tomato juice*
4 oz. veal chops
½ cup radish
½ cup lettuce
2 slices tomato (use salt substitute)
coffee, tea
Dinner *4 oz. lamb dish (see Recipe section)*
1 teaspoon mint jelly (sugarless)
coffee, tea

159

Alternate Menu #8: Combining Lamb and Veal

Breakfast *4 oz. strawberries*
2 pieces Ry-Krisp
⅓ cup cottage cheese
coffee, tea

Lunch *1 cup onion soup*
4 oz. lamb dish (see Recipe section)
coffee, tea

Dinner *½ grapefruit*
4 oz. roast veal
4 oz. carrots
4 oz. Brussels sprouts
coffee, tea

Alternate Menu #9: Combining Lamb and Liver

Breakfast *½ grapefruit*
⅓ cup cottage cheese
1 piece Melba toast
coffee, tea

Lunch *4 oz. fresh fruit cup (canned, water-packed)*
2 tablespoons liver paté or liverwurst
3 soda crackers
coffee, tea

Dinner *½ grapefruit*
4 oz. lamb dish (see Recipe section)
coffee, tea

Alternate Menu #10: Combining Lamb and Liver

Breakfast *1 orange*
1 egg, fried (Teflon pan), boiled or poached
1 piece Melba toast
coffee, tea

Lunch *8 oz. tomato soup*
4 oz. broiled lamp chops
1 tablespoon mint jelly
coffee, tea

Dinner *1 cup clear bouillon*
4 oz. liver dish (see Recipe section)
coffee, tea

Alternate Menu #11: Combining Veal and Liver

Breakfast *4 oz. applesauce*
1 boiled egg
1 piece Ry-Krisp
coffee, tea

Lunch *1 tangerine*
4 oz. grilled liver
½ cup fried onions (Teflon pan)
4 oz. broccoli
coffee, tea

Dinner *1 cup Campbell's beef soup*
4 oz.-portion veal dish (see Recipe section)
½ cup chopped eggplant
½ cup fresh beets
coffee, tea

Alternate Menu #12: Combining Veal and Liver

Breakfast *4 oz. orange juice*
1 piece whole-wheat toast
1 teaspoon butter or margarine
coffee, tea

Lunch *8 oz. onion soup*
4 oz. veal Parmigiana
coffee, tea

Dinner *4 oz. fruit cup*
6 oz. liver dish (see Recipe section)
4 oz. lettuce
2 slices tomato
coffee, tea

Keep Cool...

The alternate menus that you see above have been devised by us over a period of years, through trial and error. We have tested them on a number of our patients, all of whom were greatly amazed at how much they could eat and yet lose weight. You may feel that these menus are somewhat strange, emphasizing as they do the protein factors that we want you to ingest so as to increase your CBO time and lose that excess fat that has haunted you for so long. Don't look at them in that light; don't consider them peculiar. If you are in good health, except for the disheartening problem of being overweight, these alternate menus, like the entire Nine-Day Plan, can rid you of this depressing problem. If you happen to be under a doctor's care for any specific medical reason, you should check with him before going on any diet, not just ours.

We would like to emphasize that there is no magic to losing weight. The food plans that you will see each day in the Nine-Day Wonder Diet are based on extensive research and hard work on our part, in the hope of making the hard work on your part a little easier and very worthwhile.

Remember that you can develop odd symptoms whether you are dieting or not; don't be too quick to blame your diet for whatever peculiarities you may happen to run into while losing weight. There's no magic involved on that side of the coin either. This, of course, does not mean that if you should have any strange symptoms you should shrug them off and not bother to have them checked by your family doctor. We have found that most people feel better, not worse, on the Nine-Day Plan. Their morale is up from seeing the pounds and inches go down; they have more energy; each day becomes another certain step on the road to a gratifying success. So if you should find yourself feeling poorly, don't sit and fret about it. Get yourself checked. It shouldn't—and probably doesn't—have anything to do with the Plan, but that's no reason to ignore it. At the same time, make sure that you tell your family doctor that you are on a weight plan; that you are dieting. There should be no reason why you cannot stay on your Nine-Day Plan even if you have a cold or some other minor medical problem. One thing is certain: if you allow the excuse of getting a cold to take you off our Plan and put you back on your own—the one that got you fat to begin with—you will only reverse the process we have tried to initiate with you, weight loss, and turn it back to weight gain. Then you'll sit back and say, as you have very likely said in the past:

"That diet doesn't work." We won't let you say that about our Plan. It works. It will work for you!

RECIPES FOR ALTERNATE MENUS: DAY 5
Allowable Veal Dishes

Veal Pot Roast

2½ lbs. veal	3 tablespoons margarine
½ cup chopped onion	½ cup chopped celery
1 teaspoon salt substitute	1 clove crushed garlic
1 can Heinz tomato soup	

Brown both sides of veal in pan. Add onion, celery, sprinkle with salt substitute and garlic. Add soup and simmer until meat is tender—about two hrs. Slice, serve with gravy.

Veal Chops (not breaded)

Veal chops cut to size	2 tablespoons chopped green
1 egg	pepper
salt substitute and pepper	¼ cup margarine
½ cup skim milk	

Dip chops in beaten egg mixed with milk; you may thicken with a little flour. Brown in margarine in pan. Sprinkle with green pepper, salt substitute, ground pepper.

Veal on Skewers

veal cut in cubes	½ cup whole mushrooms
1 cup cherry tomatoes	lemon juice
2 bay leaves	1 cup small onions

Marinate the meat in lemon juice and Worcestershire sauce for several hours. Arrange on skewers, alternating the ingredients above. Broil until brown. You may have to parboil the vegetables first; it depends how well cooked you like them.

Veal Parmigiana

Purchase a Kraft frozen dinner, 13-oz. tray. You may eat 4 oz.

163

Allowable Lamb Dishes

Lamb Patties

1 lb. ground lamb
5 bacon strips
½ cup hot water
½ teaspoon salt substitute
1 bouillon cube

Shape ground meat into 4 patties; hold each with 1 strip of bacon fastened with toothpick. Grease pan with 1 teaspoon margarine. Brown patties. Pour hot bouillon into pan after patties have browned. Cover, cook over moderate heat about ½ hr. 1 patty per person. NO MORE than one for you.

Lamb Loaf

1 lb. ground lamb
1 cup flour
3 tablespoons chopped onion
1 cup bouillon
1 teaspoon salt substitute
½ cup chopped celery
2 eggs
Ehler's Garlic Pepper

Mix all ingredients and put in loaf pan. Bake in moderate oven (350°) for close to two hours.

Barbecued Lamb Ribs

lamb ribs
4 tablespoons vinegar or lemon juice
2 teaspoons salt substitute
2 tablespoons Worcestershire sauce
1 cup chopped onion
½ tablespoon mustard
½ cup chopped celery
Cayenne pepper

Bake ribs in shallow pan for half an hour at 350°. Sauté onion, add other ingredients, simmer for five to ten minutes. Pour over ribs and bake one hour more. Baste with sauce.

Roast Leg or Shoulder of Lamb

This is one of our favorite dishes. You can use either with stuffing provided it has been boned and a pocket has been cut. Rub the meat with garlic and salt substitute after making sure it is as dry as possible. It can be stuffed with chopped-meat stuffing or a celery-bread stuffing that you can eat provided you take no more than half a cup. The idea is to eat more meat than anything else.

164

4 lb. lamb shoulder
3 teaspoons salt substitute
1 cup chopped celery
2 eggs
½ cup chopped onion

¼ teaspoon curry powder
¼ teaspoon paprika
2 lbs. chopped chuck
½ cup skim milk
2 tablespoons Wesson oil

Combine ingredients. Beat egg yolks after separating from whites. Mix all ingredients with chopped chuck. Milk should not be left over in the bowl; make sure it combines completely with the meat. Pack the stuffing into the pocket and sew or skewer it closed. Bake at 350° for about forty minutes per pound. When lamb is done, take from oven, let stand at room temperature for twenty minutes. (This locks in the flavor.) With the chopped meat stuffing you can eat as much as anyone else. Quite delicious—we've gotten many compliments on this dish; you should too.

Allowable Liver Dishes

Liver and Onions
1 lb. liver
2 tablespoons margarine
pepper

2 cups sliced onions
salt substitute
garlic salt

Fry onions in hot margarine, sprinkle with condiments. Add liver slices, cook five to eight minutes until done to taste. You may eat this rare or well done; it will make no difference to your weight loss, despite what people may tell you.

Chopped Liver
1 lb. liver
2 tablespoons chicken fat or
   lard)
salt substitute

hard-boiled eggs
chopped onion
pepper

Boil liver and let cool. Grind to coarse consistency (do not make it into a paste). Do the same with the eggs and onion. Salt and pepper to taste. Add chicken fat after mixing ingredients to get proper consistency. Serve on bed of lettuce or individual pieces of Ry-Krisp. You may garnish with parsley sprigs.

Spanish Liver

1 lb. sliced liver	1 bay leaf
½ cup chopped onion	½ cup salad oil
1 teaspoon salt substitute	3 tablespoons lemon juice
1 tablespoon ketchup	1 cup Heinz tomato soup

Rub slices of liver with chopped onion, allowing pieces of onion to imbed in liver. Mix oil and lemon juice as a marinade; place liver slices in this for one to two hours. Cut liver into cubes, add bay leaf, salt substitute (or pepper) and simmer in tomato soup until tender. Before serving remove bay leaf, add ketchup, allow to simmer five more minutes. Serve with paprika.

Allowable Beef Dishes

Brisket

3 lbs. beef brisket	1 carrot
2 tablespoons cooking oil	½ cup chopped celery
1 sliced onion	salt substitute
½ cup vinegar	pepper

Brown slices of brisket in hot butter; add other ingredients to pan; cover and simmer for two hours.

Goulash

leftover brisket or roast beef	1 can tomatoes
small onions	1 cup water
2 tablespoons butter	salt substitute

Dice meat into pan, add water and tomatoes and cook for thirty minutes. Boil onions in water till tender, then add; or sauté in butter, fry and add to meat. Season from zero-calorie list.

Beef Pot Roast

3 lbs. chuck meat	salt substitute
pepper	3 tablespoons Crisco or Wesson
hot water	oil

Make sure meat is dry; rub with salt and pepper. Heat oil in pot or heavy skillet. Brown meat on all sides, add water to cover and simmer for two hours, adding water as necessary. Transfer to oven at 300° till tender. You may use the liquid in the pot or skillet as

166

gravy. Do NOT thicken; use as is. You may add onions and carrots to this meat when it is simmering in pot; make sure the water level is sufficient.

Breakfast Steak

2 lbs. round steak	*3 tablespoons oil*
flour	*Heinz tomato soup*
salt substitute	*pepper*

Sprinkle meat with flour, salt substitute and pepper; brown in hot oil, pour in tomato soup and bake in hot oven (400°) for half an hour or brown in skillet.

Remember...

You may NOT substitute any part of one alternate menu for another.

You may NOT substitute any part of an alternate menu for the Basic Menu.

The same holds true for the alternate menus as for the Basic Menu so far as times of eating are concerned. You must try to eat something during these periods even if you are not hungry. We have tried to arrange menus that have something for everyone. Of course, you must not eat *more* than is allowed; nor will you have any snacks between meals other than your apricots and skim milk. Once the eating time zone is over, eat nothing except the permitted snack until the next eating zone (the next meal) has arrived. Your proper CBO is dependent on all things going as we have calculated as exactly as is possible.

ACT LIKE A WINNER AND YOU'LL BE A LOSER

There are people who are never satisfied. Don't be one of them. You will find that today you should have every cause for satisfaction. This is the day you will be weighing yourself for the first time since starting the Plan. However, don't feel that just because you've done everything you were supposed to a miracle will occur today and you will have lost all your excess weight.

You may feel this way because of the two fast days you've just accomplished. But we want you to realize that, while it is possible for you to find yourself at normal weight today (this could happen, as we mentioned earlier, depending on how much weight you had to lose), chances are that you will not. Indeed, you may find you've lost only a couple of pounds. It is unlikely that you will have lost only two pounds up to this point if you've followed all instructions, but, as we keep pointing out, everyone is different, and everyone loses weight at a different rate of speed. Strangely enough, the individual who has lost just two pounds up to the first weighing is not usually the one who does all the complaining. Such people usually tell us, "I lost two pounds by the fifth day of your plan, but it took me a month on other plans to lose that much. It is worth it to me to continue with this plan, to persevere and lose more weight." This is the type of individual who will end up losing eight or more pounds on the completed cycle, will be very excited about this success and will be ready to do it again and lose more weight.

The individual who gets upset after weighing is more than likely someone who has lost four or five pounds—and is still bitterly unsatisfied. What, five pounds already gone by the fifth day? A pound a day and more to come? That's great, we think. But not this individual. He says: "I should have lost more!"

That remark is a putdown; that person is a loser. Not a weight loser, just a loser. The other people—the ones who lose two pounds and go on to finish the job—are the ultimate winners, even though their weight loss has not been immediately so great.

Don't be a loser. Don't think like one. Never say, "I should have lost more." It's a bit late for you to be making the rules. Who says you should have lost more? Only you. By that token you never should have gotten fat. "I should have lost more" is a phrase that reflects lack of confidence in yourself, a lack of confidence that is all too ready to burst forth and spread to whatever you happen to be doing. It is especially good at destroying your diet. It will load you with stress. Most people have enough stress in their lives without looking for more. As we pointed out earlier, stress—the opposite of relaxation—will make you eat more. That will make you a loser all right, but not the kind you want to be.

Look at the winners. Look at the people who are successful in life: the executives, the jet-setters, the wealthy and powerful. By and large, most of them are slim. How come? Well, as one of our patients who works for a large company put it: "My boss is thin. He never gets heartburn; he gives it."

At a meeting we attended some years ago, one of the speakers said the same thing in a slightly different way. He said that overweight in this country is a class phenomenon. He didn't mean that it's classy to be fat, but that overweight is not an equal opportunity employer—there are a great many social and economic factors that influence it. You might think, then, that it would be the wealthier among us—those who can easily afford all the food they want—who would be fat, and that the rest of us—to whom food is a great expense—would be thin.

Just the opposite.

Overweight, and especially obesity, is almost absent in the upper classes—especially among women. In the classic phrase, it is impossible to be too rich or too thin. We middle-class and poor people are mainly the ones who get fat; we who can ill afford to do so from every aspect. We are the ones who make food such a status symbol, and invest it with overtones of hospitality so that as soon as someone walks in our door there must be food on the table to offer and to share. We idolize food and we sacrifice burnt offerings to our stomach (no reflection on any of our readers' cooking abilities).

But the very wealthy, surrounded by food, have other status symbols. Many such people with whom we have discussed this feel that it is a measure of their power to turn away from the temptation of overeating. They like to win challenges.

You, like them, can be a winner in this regard. There are several things you can do to play the winning game.

1. Find some way to pass your stresses along. Take the time to seek out a method of doing this that is custom-made for you. We aren't advising that you go home, kick the dog and beat up your spouse. But you must develop some activity that will allow your stress runoff time. It may be a sport; it may be a hobby. Develop it now, while you are losing weight, so that when you get down to ideal weight you will be able to stay there.

2. Use your relaxation techniques each day as we have outlined them. Develop others. This must continue even when you are no

169

longer overweight. Make relaxation as much a habit as your daily exercising. This way, when you get down to "fighting trim" you'll have fewer problems to fight.

3. Recognize the occasions of "ritual overeating": the family gatherings, the births, the marriages, the funerals. Don't automatically start to use food as a tool for socializing, as a gesture of sympathy or celebration.

4. Don't let food take on exaggerated importance. Think how the refrigerator is replacing the hearth as a symbol of your home. "As soon as I get in my house, I head for the refrigerator. It's as if the front door was that door," one woman confessed. She was so horrified to discover that this was all her home meant to her that she determined to stop doing it.

5. Don't put yourself in the hands of amateurs or quacks at a time when you are seriously interested in losing weight. Your friends and relatives may well qualify as such. Stay with a proven plan; stay with experts. You deserve the best; with our Nine-Day Plan, that's what you are getting.

6. Take every occasion one at a time. Don't attempt to handle everything at once. This is why we've worked out the Nine-Day Wonder Diet for you one day at a time. It is no accident that each day is different. Each day of your life is different. You live one day at a time; you lose weight one day at a time.

The techniques you learn in losing weight will stand you in good stead in other aspects of your life. It is a measure of character to lose weight and get to be the person you always knew you were but that few others realized you could be. Many of the people we have treated found that losing weight made them more desirable even in terms of their careers. One example may serve out of hundreds. Joseph W. worked in a large supermarket in a minor position. With our help he lost eighty-five pounds. Today he is manager of the store—a situation that came about through his loss of weight. His boss told him: "Joe, if you can do that job, you can do any job."

You, too, can feel competent and in control.

That's what being a winner means.

9

THURSDAY: THE FOWL AND FISH DAY

We'd like to take a moment or two here to do a little explaining. Don't worry, we aren't going to hold you up from proceeding with your diet for long. However, there are certain things you should know. We've told you that we realize you are basically interested in results, not theory. That still holds true, but we feel it is important that you understand a bit more about the facts of what we are doing.

A LITTLE SCIENCE

Yesterday we went through a twenty-four-hour period that was based on what we like to call "full" or "heavy" protein. This consisted of meats—specifically beef—as well as veal, lamb and liver. The Basic Menu stressed these meats through the day; alternatives revolved around them for the main meal and at least one other. Many people have told us (before they really tried it) that they couldn't eat meat three times a day. If you are one of these individuals, use one of the alternate menus. We don't want to force you into a pattern you aren't ready for; perhaps the alternate menu here will help you work up to using the Basic Menu next cycle. It's perfectly all right to sneak up on success.

How does "full" protein dieting take pounds off you? If you

understand this you might be more apt to follow closely what we want you to do. First of all, what is protein? This substance is one of the three kinds of food your body needs to stay alive and healthy. It uses protein to rebuild itself, to replace used-up blood cells as well as other portions of its fabric that keep breaking down and need repair; it uses it, of course, for growth. So protein is actually the body's building blocks. Only in times of extreme emergency does the body use it for fuel. At all other times it uses fats and carbohydrates; protein is burned only in cases of starvation. Protein means "many-shaped" or "many-faceted," and these long chemical strands are just that. They branch and rebranch all over the place like lines of railroad cars hooked together at various angles. These railroad cars are amino acids; the body requires certain of them to stay alive and healthy. We are going to have you utilize them not only to be healthier, but to lose weight. It works like this:

HOW PROTEIN DIETING TAKES OFF POUNDS FAST

1. First of all, protein is filling—and it is filling partly because it is chewable. It is also highly nutritious; therefore, when you eat it, you will not be craving other items as a stopgap to your hunger. Why, then, don't more people utilize it as such? Because the food industry doesn't want you to; their profit comes from items that return to them more money per ounce than does protein, which is fairly expensive all around. Also, the business of the food industry is to get you to eat. To eat much more than you really want to—hence all the money they spend on advertising. Would anyone really have to spend money to impel you to eat if you were really hungry? Of course not. But the food industry does it all the time. And what do they do it with? Not protein, which, as we have said, does not return to them the profit they would like to have, but with carbohydrates, which actually make you hungrier. So it becomes a continuous cycle. You can break this cycle with protein dieting, a technique we initiated for you yesterday and which we will further implement today.

2. Protein takes fat from your body. How? Think of it this way. When you eat carbohydrate—most people think of sugar in this

172

regard, and it is indeed the principal carbohydrate that gets you fat—these materials go easily into the absorptive lining of your intestinal tract. Very little energy need be expended by your body to take them into the bloodstream, and they are themselves stored as energy—fat—against such time as they may be needed. But when you eat protein, it takes a considerable amount of energy for the body to break down and absorb these stubborn chain-linked molecules. Yet the body *must* take them into the bloodstream, so it must spend whatever energy is necessary in order to do this. Where does this energy come from? From the body burning your fat. Each pound that it burns releases 3,500 calories of energy. Therefore, the more protein you eat, the more fat—and weight—you are likely to lose.

3. Wait a minute, you may say here. If I lose fat because it is burned up from the protein I am eating, won't my weight stay just as it was from the added weight of the ingested protein? Good question. Someone in our lectures always asks it. But no, your weight won't stay the same from ingested protein because there is a big difference in the way your body treats protein as opposed to the way it treats carbohydrate. It stores carbohydrate as fat, but it will not store protein as fat. In fact, it will not store protein at all. It gets rid of what it cannot immediately use. If it treated carbohydrate that way, no one in the world would ever have a problem with over-weight. But you must understand that the one thing your body does store is carbohydrate—fat—as a sort of banked energy against a time of famine. Time passes, the famine doesn't arrive... but you keep eating and your body keeps storing. It won't store water, it won't store vitamins, it won't store minerals, hormones, protein— only carbohydrate. Many people get confused by this. They think that because their bodies store fat, if they eat fat they will get fat. Not true. Your body doesn't really store fat—not the fat that you eat as such. In fact, if you ate only fat you'd get thin, because it costs your body more energy to absorb the fat you've eaten than the fat itself supplies; twice as much, in fact. Of course, if you ate that much fat, you would also get sick, and we certainly do not recommend it.

4. There is no water retention associated with eating protein. When you take in a great amount of carbohydrate foods (a carbohydrate food being, among other things, anything that grows in the ground that is edible), you take in a great deal of "lock-in" water as well. We call it this because as your body deposits fat from the carbohydrates in the fat depots, it deposits quite a bit of water as well. You will not be able to get rid of this water until you burn a certain amount of fat. The rule of thumb is: lose a pound of fat, lose a pound of water. But because protein food is not stored by the body, water retention through ingesting it is minimal—provided that you watch the salt, of course.

5. Protein eating helps you accomplish a "different" pattern of food ingestion, especially the way in which we've worked it out for you. That's good. A break from your previous eating habits is essential to get you to lose weight, and especially to get you to lose inches. Most of your Nine-Day Plan has been calculated to accomplish this. Interestingly, many people tell us that they find the protein days the most exciting—even more so than the fast days. This new style of eating points up the things you've been doing to yourself that get you into trouble. For instance, that extra piece of toast in the morning. We know it isn't that piece of toast that has gotten you fat—it's the state of mind that goes with it, that chooses this item over others that will take the inches off. Yet, you think: "I'll get away with it." How many times have you gone to eat something that has always proved disastrous before and nevertheless still thought this? And you do get away with it—it will go with you as part of your fat collection. Eat protein and you'll *do* away with it.

TWO TYPES OF PROTEIN

Yesterday was the first protein day. You were given in the Basic Menu what we like to call "full" or "heavy" protein foods to choose from. These were mainly beef items or substances fairly similar in CBO time. Today you will be eating the "lighter" proteins: various fish and fowl that we have found to be the best for the purpose. And what is this purpose? Not only to drop pounds, but inches as well. Yes, it has been our experience that varying the protein foods from "heavy" to "light" not only helps your weight come off more swiftly, but gives your body a chance to draw some of its fat from between the muscle fibers, thus actually helping you lose inches more efficiently: those bulges will go down. It is interesting how many of our patients learned this little technique for themselves while on some other plan that didn't include it. We have been working with it for years, placing patients on "test periods" during which time they ate mostly fish and fowl, and lost amazing numbers of inches (some women going down three dress sizes) where they had the most to lose. In your Nine-Day Plan we have incorporated this technique among the other portions of the plan in such a way as to give it maximum effect in a short amount of time—thus eliminating the boredom that could come from weeks of eating this way only. Two days, if you follow instructions, can be enough to make great changes in your weight *placement,* to say nothing of actual loss.

WHAT YOU WILL EAT TODAY

1. Those eight glasses of water.

2. Your multivitamin-mineral tablet.

3. Your "total contentment" pill (if you so choose—again, remember to drink your water with this).

4. You may have coffee or tea at will; ⅓ teaspoon of nondairy creamer is allowed.

5. You may have the following vegetable snacks between meals today: either one carrot and half a medium apple or two celery stalks and a whole orange. You do not HAVE to eat these items; if you choose to do so, do not mix or interchange the two groups. YOU MAY NOT EAT ANYTHING AFTER TEN P.M.

6. You may have up to two cans of diet soda today. Do not drink both cans at once; it is much better if you divide them over the day.

PREPARING TODAY'S FOOD

You may roast, boil, broil, barbecue or pan-fry (using a Teflon pan) today's foods. No deep-fat frying or breading is allowed. You may use a small amount of butter sauce with your lobster or crab legs provided there is no salt in the butter. DO NOT USE SALT at all today. Canned fish must be water-packed today or not used.

BASIC MENU: DAY 6

Breakfast ½ cup tomato juice
2 oz. canned tuna fish
2 pieces Ry-Krisp
coffee, tea

Lunch 1 cup clear bouillon
4 oz. brook trout
½ cup lettuce
½ cup tomato
½ cup celery
wine vinegar
coffee, tea

Dinner 6 oz. turkey breast (that part of the turkey only)
½ cup endive or lettuce
½ cup green pepper
½ cup cucumber
½ cup mushrooms
coffee, tea

We want to make it clear that, on this day as on all the others, following the Basic Menu will likely give you the most substantial weight loss for the day. However, while we have found this true for the majority of our patients, there *were* others who lost more on one of the alternate plans. That is why w provide them; as we keep pointing out, individual variation is a prime factor when dealing with human beings. We recognize the fact that none of you is a machine and that each of your bodies, while being a large chemical factory for food, operates according to quirks of its own with various degrees of efficiency. However, whether you are following the Basic Menu or one of the alternates, if for some reason the Basic Menu doesn't appeal to you, the same rules of eating prevail. You may eat less than but *no more* than is allowed. You must sit at the table to eat, and you may do so only during the times allowed. These are the same times as yesterday. If you miss a particular time, you miss the meal. There is no carrying over of calories you do not eat at one meal to the next one.

ALTERNATE MENUS TO TODAY'S PLAN
Alternate Menu #1: (Combining Fish, Seafood and Fowl)
Breakfast ½ grapefruit
  2 oz. canned salmon (water-packed only)
  1 piece Ry-Krisp
  tea, coffee
Lunch 4 oz. shrimp
  6 stalks fresh or canned asparagus
  ½ cup mushrooms
  ½ cup lettuce
  ½ cup cucumbers
  seasoning to taste from zero-calorie list
  coffee, tea, diet soda
Dinner ½ cup tomato juice
  6 oz. breast of chicken
  ½ cup green peppers (raw or cooked)
  ½ cup mushrooms (raw or cooked*)
  coffee, tea

*The peppers and mushrooms may be fried only in a Teflon pan; that is, without oil or butter.

Alternate Menu #2: (Combining Fish, Seafood and Fowl
Breakfast 2 oz. smoked salmon (Vita)*
  3 pieces Ry-Krisp
  coffee, tea

*You may also use fresh smoked salmon—preferably the Nova Scotia variety, which is the less salty of the two types available.

Lunch 4 oz. crabmeat cocktail (see Recipe section)
  seasonings from zero-calorie list
  1 cup lettuce
  ½ cup radishes
  ½ cup cucumbers
  coffee, tea

Dinner 1 cup clear soup
4 oz. Chicken Cacciatore
½ cup plain boiled rice
½ cup onion as side dish
½ cup mushrooms
2 slices tomato
coffee, tea

Alternate Menu #3: Combining Fish, Seafood and Fowl

Breakfast ½ grapefruit
4 oz. pickled herring (no sour cream; Vita brand only)
3 pieces Ry-Krisp
coffee, tea
Lunch 8 oz. Manhattan-style clam chowder, either canned or fresh

OR

6 oz. New England-style clam chowder, canned or fresh
4 saltine crackers (Keebler or Premium)
coffee, tea
Dinner 1 cup bouillon or ½ cup tomato juice
4 oz.-portion stuffed turkey (see Recipe section)
½ cup cucumbers
6 asparagus stalks
coffee, tea

Alternate Menu #4: Combining Seafood, Fowl and Wine

We call this the "show biz special," since many of our patients in that line of work, when called upon to lose weight quickly to get a desired part in a play or opera, have used this variation to slim down rapidly and still eat.

Breakfast 6 oz. orange juice, either fresh or frozen
2 oz. black or red caviar
½ oz. chopped onion
½ oz. chopped egg yolk
3 pieces Ry-Krisp, broken up
¼ oz.-glass champagne

178

Lunch *1 doz. clams with horseradish sauce or plain with lemon
juice (clams must be raw)*
OR
4 oz. cold lobster salad (see Recipe section)
Dinner *4 oz. coq au vin*
½ cup green peppers
½ cup mushrooms
*½ cup corn, fresh or canned (if fresh, 1 small ear, and use
salt substitute)*
2 oz. domestic Burgundy (Taylor Wine)
coffee, tea

An alternative to this alternate menu is to repeat the breakfast
menu at dinner time. This menu can also be utilized without the
wine portions if you so wish. If you like caviar and raw seafood, this
may just be for you. Obviously you need not buy the expensive
name-brand caviars; you can find good, inexpensive ones in your
local food store. Vita is one brand that we ourselves have used; it is
excellent and not expensive.

Alternate Menu #5: Combining Fish and Seafood

Breakfast *4 oz. orange juice, fresh or canned*
4 oz. grilled brook trout
2 slices fresh tomato
½ cup onion
coffee, tea
Lunch *1 doz. clams or oysters raw or cooked (see Recipe section)*
1 4 oz.-glass beer
OR
8 oz. Manhattan-style clam chowder
2 sesame crackers
coffee, tea
Dinner *1 cup consommé*
6 oz. red snapper in tomato sauce
½ cup celery
½ cup green peppers
coffee, tea

Alternate Menu #6: Combining Fish and Seafood

Breakfast 2 oz. canned tuna fish (water-packed)
          2 pieces Ry-Krisp
          seasoning from zero-calorie list
          coffee, tea

Lunch ½ cup tomato juice
          8 oz. portion Spanish Shrimp (see Recipe section)
          3 Ritz crackers
          coffee, tea

Dinner ½ cup endive
          ½ cup escarole
          ½ cup green peppers
          2 lettuce leaves
          6 oz. baked striped bass
          coffee, tea

Alternate Menu #7: Combining Fish and Seafood

Breakfast 6 oz. orange juice
          2 oz. smoked whitefish
          coffee, tea

Lunch 6 oz. fried or broiled scallops
          seasoning from zero-calorie list
          ½ cup grapefruit and orange sections
          ½ cup lettuce
          coffee, tea

Dinner 6 oz. codfish cakes (see Recipe section)
          1 medium potato
          coffee, tea

Alternate Menu #8: Combining Fish and Seafood
Two Meals Only

Breakfast 1 medium orange
          2 pieces Melba toast
          1 boiled or poached egg
          coffee, tea

Lunch *4 oz. shrimp cocktail*
sauce from zero-calorie list
½ cup lettuce
½ cup celery
½ cup tomato
coffee, tea
Dinner *½ cup tomato juice*
½ cup green peppers
½ cup onion
½ cup mushrooms
8 oz. flounder, pan-fried or broiled
1 fresh ear of corn (or ½ cup canned corn)
coffee, tea

Alternate Menu #9: Combining Fish and Seafood Two Meals Only

Breakfast *3 oz. orange juice*
2 pieces Ry-Krisp
⅓ cup cottage cheese
coffee, tea
Lunch *4 oz. sardines in tomato sauce*
½ cup green peppers
½ cup lettuce
½ cup onion
½ cup radishes
tea, coffee, diet soda
Dinner *4 oz. tomato juice (½ cup)*
8 oz. lobster (see Recipe section)
coffee, tea

Alternate Menu #10: Fish Only

Breakfast *4 oz. orange juice*
4 oz. canned tuna fish
seasoning from zero-calorie list
coffee, tea
Lunch *6 oz. grilled flounder*
½ cup lettuce
½ cup green peppers

lemon wedge
½ cup onion
½ cup mushrooms
coffee, tea
Dinner 1 cup clear bouillon
6 oz. codfish cakes (you may substitute haddock, bass or
pike)
½ cup cauliflower or broccoli
coffee, tea

Alternate Menu #11: Fish Only

Breakfast 8 oz. tomato juice or ½ grapefruit
4 oz. broiled flounder
lemon wedge
2 pieces Melba toast
coffee, tea
Lunch ½ melon (medium cantaloupe)
6 oz. broiled mackerel or lake trout
lemon wedge
½ cup onion
½ cup mushrooms
coffee, tea
Dinner 4 oz. pineapple (fresh or canned, water-packed) or 1
medium nectarine
8 oz. haddock dish (see Recipe section)
OR
4 oz. swordfish grilled, in which case you may add the
following:
6 stalks fresh or canned asparagus
½ cup green peppers
coffee, tea

Alternate Menu #12: Seafood Only

Breakfast ½ grapefruit
4 oz. crabmeat patties (see Recipe section)
2 pieces Melba toast
coffee, tea

Lunch   1 two-inch wedge honeydew melon
6 oz. shrimp cocktail (includes cocktail sauce)
2 lettuce leaves
coffee, tea
Dinner   ½ cup fruit salad
8 oz. portion oven-fried shrimp
coffee, tea

Alternate Menu #13: Seafood Only

You have to really be crazy about seafood to go for this one. The two of us happen to be, and so we are including this for those of you who feel the same way. If shellfish is not your dish, just skip this alternate.

Breakfast   6 oz. Clamato juice
6 oz. shrimp cocktail (includes sauce)
½ cup lettuce
6 oysterettes
coffee, tea
Lunch   8 oz. Manhattan-style clam chowder
2 doz. raw clams or mixed clams and oysters (2 doz. total).
Lemon juice or horseradish sauce only
3 Ritz crackers
coffee, tea
Dinner   4 oz. applesauce
6 oz. broiled soft-shell crabs (see Recipe section)
coffee, tea

Alternate Menu #14: Fowl Only

Breakfast   4 oz. orange juice
2 eggs done in different ways: perhaps 1 fried (no butter or margarine), 1 scrambled or poached.
2 pieces Ry-Krisp
coffee, tea
Lunch   6 oz. chicken salad (see Recipe section)
2 pieces Ry-Krisp
coffee, tea

Dinner 1 cup clear soup (unsalted)
4 oz. portion roast duck
coffee, tea

Alternate Menu #15: Fowl Only
Breakfast ½ grapefruit
1 medium egg (hard-boiled or poached)
2 pieces Ry-Krisp
coffee, tea
Lunch 1 medium orange or pot cheese
6 oz. broiled chicken breast
½ cup carrots
½ cup eggplant
coffee, tea
Dinner ½ cup strawberries
6 oz. turkey dish (see Recipe section)
coffee, tea

Alternate Menu #16: Fowl and Dairy
Breakfast 4 oz. apple juice
1 fried egg (no butter or margarine)
2 pieces Melba toast
1 oz. cream cheese
coffee, tea
Lunch 1 cup skim milk or buttermilk
3 slices Oscar Mayer turkey breast lunch meat
½ cup lettuce
½ cup green peppers
coffee, tea
Dinner ½ cup fruit cocktail, fresh or water-packed
6 oz. portion chicken fricassee
OR
4 oz. portion chicken fricassee
⅓ cup cottage or pot cheese
coffee, tea

RECIPES FOR DAY 6
Allowable Chicken Dishes

Broiled Chicken Livers

chicken livers	pepper
salt substitute	lettuce leaves
green pepper	garlic powder
melted butter (1 tablespoon)	chopped chives or parsley

Place livers on broiler rack about four inches below heat source. Cook about four minutes per side before checking; after that watch very carefully or they will get too well done. We prefer chicken livers medium-rare. (Many people are only acquainted with liver in a leathery state. This is unfortunate.) Serve sprinkled with chopped chives or parsley. Lettuce leaves may be used as a base. You may include fried onions with this dish provided you fry them only in a Teflon pan. No additional butter should be added to this recipe.

Roast Chicken

chicken parts	Lawry's Seasoned Pepper
garlic clove	onions
paprika	celery and carrots

Dry the chicken and rub the seasonings well into the skin. You will be able to eat the skin, so make it tasty. Place in roasting pan and put under broiler until skin is crisp. Add vegetables to the pan. Sprinkle paprika over the chicken once again before serving.

French Chicken

broiler parts	tarragon leaves
minced shallots	dry white wine

Roll chicken parts in either fresh or dry tarragon leaves, marinate in dry white wine with three to four minced shallots for approximately one hour. Preheat oven and broil until tender, basting every so often with the marinade. Serve gravy separately—don't waste it. You may use the gravy sparingly. It is to be used for flavoring, not for drinking.

Barbecued Chicken

a broiler in quarters
melted butter
barbecue sauce

salt and pepper to taste
(salt substitute)

Broil the chicken, placing the parts five to eight inches from the heat. Cook about half an hour, turning often. Brush the parts for the last ten minutes with plenty of barbecue sauce.

Spanish Chicken

2 or 3 lb. fryer
½ cup chopped onion
½ cup chopped green peppers
1 can Heinz tomato soup
½ cup sliced stuffed olives
½ cup sautéed mushrooms

¼ cup olive oil
1 clove garlic
¼ cup hot spiced peppers
1 cup chopped, peeled, seeded
   tomatoes

Brown chicken in hot olive oil and place in casserole. In the pan add onion, peppers, garlic, tomatoes and tomato soup. Pour over chicken in casserole. Bake for one hour at 350°. Add mushrooms and olives a few minutes before removing chicken from casserole to serve. Delicious!

Chicken Cacciatore

Chicken parts
olive oil
tomato paste
salt substitute
bouillon
allspice
sliced mushrooms

flour
chopped shallots
white wine
Lawry's seasoned pepper
bay leaf
tarragon

Sprinkle pieces of chicken with flour, then brown gently in a skillet with hot olive oil; gradually add chopped shallots and then all the other ingredients. Cover the pan and let all simmer for about one hour.

186

Stuffed Turkey

turkey, whole	chopped meat
tomato paste	egg yolks, beaten
barbecue sauce	chopped celery
chopped onion	salt substitute
Lawry's seasoned pepper	paprika
¾ cup butter (approximately)	

3 cups of stuffing should fill a ten-pound bird. Mix chopped meat, egg yolks, onion and celery together. Add seasonings and barbecue sauce to taste. Stuff mixture into bird and sew or skewer closed. Preheat oven to 450°; reduce to 350° when placing bird inside. Use a rack and allow about twenty-five minutes per pound to cook. Baste with melted butter constantly. One way to make sure that your bird will be moist is to wrap it in cheesecloth. The interstices of the cloth will hold the basting material fairly evenly over the skin. CAUTION: Do not pack your stuffing too tightly. You will find that there is plenty of room to keep pushing more in, but if you do this the stuffing will not cook properly. We have found that just a little more pressure than gravity gives the best result.

Coq au Vin

3-4 lb. roasting chicken	sherry
½ cup each chopped onions,	olive oil
celery, carrots, green pepper	Lawry's Seasoned Pepper
1 clove chopped garlic	1 tablespoon flour
salt substitute to taste	

Brown chicken in hot oil in a casserole while sautéeing vegetables in a pan. Add to the chicken bay leaf and marjoram; you may add sliced mushrooms. Pour in sherry. Then pour vegetables over chicken. Use flour to thicken gravy.

Allowable Seafood Dishes

Chinese Shrimp

1½ lbs. raw shrimp	scallions
vegetable oil	bouillon
sliced ginger or ginger powder	Lawry's Seasoned Pepper
salt substitute	1 egg
cornstarch	soy sauce

Mix together starch and soy sauce in a little water; set aside. Place in pan oil, salt, pepper, ginger and garlic. Heat for one minute; add shrimp and stir for about two minutes. Add bouillon, simmer five minutes. Then add cornstarch and soy sauce and mix until juice thickens smoothly. Add beaten eggs and scallions. Do not allow mixture to boil.

Spanish Shrimp

1½ lbs. raw shrimp	ginger powder
2 bell peppers, sliced	Lawry's Seasoned Pepper
salt substitute	1 cup bouillon or vegetable
1 clove crushed garlic, fresh	stock
1 cup fresh or canned tomatoes	1 tablespoon cornstarch
soy sauce to taste	2 chopped scallions
1 tablespoon sliced ginger or	olive oil

Slice bell peppers and parboil. Chop tomatoes. Cut shrimp along the back but not completely through the body. Place oil, salt, pepper, ginger and garlic in hot pan; add shrimp. Sauté for two to three minutes, then add bouillon and peppers. Mix well, cook at medium heat for about ten minutes. Then add starch, tomatoes and scallions. Stir till juice thickens, then serve.

Crabmeat Cocktail

You may use canned crabmeat (Bumble Bee brand), which comes in a 7½-ounce can. Eat somewhat less than half of it. Arrange as you would a shrimp cocktail on a bed of lettuce with horseradish or cocktail sauce. If you want to use fresh crabmeat you may certainly do this according to the amount given in the menu. Cold lobster salad is done in the same way.

Stuffed Lobster Tails

4 frozen lobster tails   chopped parsley
1 onion, chopped fine   1½ cups bread crumbs
1 mashed fresh garlic clove   olive oil

After thawing the tails, cut underside of shell away. Broil at medium heat for about five minutes, then turn cut side up and cover with stuffing made by mix of onion, garlic, parsley, bread crumbs and oil. Broil for about another ten minutes, checking constantly for the last five minutes.

Broiled Lobster

Treat as above, except that you may eat all the edible portions including the tail. Use a considerable amount of lemon juice. Be careful with the butter sauce, using the following scale of proportions of lobster to sauce: For a 4-oz. portion of lobster you may use 1 tablespoon of butter sauce; for a 6-oz. portion, 2 teaspoons butter sauce; and for an 8-oz. portion, no more than 1 teaspoon of butter sauce. If you dilute the butter sauce you are allowed with plenty of lemon juice or other seasonings from the zero-calorie list, you will find that you can extend the allowed amounts sufficiently to flavor the largest amount of lobster on the menu.

Oysters Rockefeller

We like to leave the butter out of this dish and cover the raw oysters with some raw chopped onion, lemon juice and chopped parsley. Sprinkle with a minimum of bread crumbs and a little Worcestershire sauce. Imbed the oysters (in the bottom shell) in rock salt, bake for about ten minutes at 400°, then broil till brown. You may sprinkle some bacon bits onto the oysters if you wish, but we suggest that you do not wrap those oysters you have earmarked for yourself with bacon strips, as is usually done with this dish. That has not been allowed for in calculating your CBO, nor has the spinach that is sometimes served with these oysters. It is simple enough to remove the spinach and the bacon if you are at a party where these are being served. Of the two, it is more important that the bacon not be eaten.

Steamed Clams

The thing to watch out for here is the salt; this means that you can dip the steamers in the broth but do not drink it. Remember not to oversteam your clams; overcooking makes clams tough. Again, this is a dish you can use a lot of lemon on. If you like melted butter with your steamers, you may have it in roughly the same proportion as you used for your lobster: calculate 1 tablespoon butter sauce per one dozen clams, 2 teaspoons sauce per two dozen clams and 1 teaspoon per three dozen (the maximum). Use your zero-calorie list to help spread the butter out and make it go further.

Broiled Clams

Preheat the broiler and put in cherrystone clams on the half shell. Cover each with a dash of Worcestershire sauce, lemon juice and chopped parsley. Broil for about five minutes.

Broiled Soft-Shell Crabs

These are also a perfect seafood for your diet. After preheating the broiler, mix ¼ cup of butter with three tablespoons of lemon juice, salt substitute and Lawry's Seasoned Pepper. Roll your crabs in this, and broil for five or six minutes.

Crabmeat Patties

Melt butter in a saucepan and put in some pieces of garlic. Add flour and milk until sauce is thick; then put in salt substitute, pepper and Worcestershire sauce. Add a small amount of bread crumbs to half the sauce as well as to crabmeat. (We suggest Bumble Bee canned variety if you are not going to use fresh.) Mix, put in refrigerator to chill. Shape into small patties, dip each into a beaten egg. Fry in Teflon pan and serve with reheated remaining sauce. CAUTION: WATCH THE BREAD CRUMBS.

Allowable Fish Dishes

Grilled Swordfish

2 tablespoons butter
1 tablespoon lemon juice
salt substitute to taste
lemon wedges
1 tablespoon tarragon leaves
(fresh or dry)
1 swordfish steak
black pepper to taste
oil

Charcoal broiling this fish is really the way to go. Melt butter, add lemon juice and tarragon. Sprinkle steak with salt and pepper. Brush oil over hot grill and put on steak. It is important you do this or the unoiled grill will tear the steak. Brush steak with melted butter; broil about eight minutes on each side. Swordfish calls for a lot of butter, which is the reason only four ounces of it are allowed. But done this way it will be a superb four ounces. Serve with lemon wedges surrounding.

Stuffed Haddock

½ cup chopped onion
½ cup chopped mushrooms
oil
salt substitute
haddock fillets
peeled sliced tomatoes
½ cup chopped celery
½ cup chopped green pepper
bread crumbs (½ cup)
pepper
lemon juice

After preheating the oven to 375°, sauté the onion, celery and mushrooms in the oil; after a few minutes add the salt substitute and pepper. Place the haddock fillets in a baking dish, sprinkle these with plenty of lemon juice and spread the onion mix over them. Cover all this with the peeled sliced tomatoes and bake for approximately half an hour to forty minutes.

Codfish Cakes

½ pound unsalted codfish
1 small potato
vegetable oil
½ cup chopped onion

Cut fish into small pieces and cook with small pieces of potato until tender. After draining off the water, mash up potato, oil, onion and codfish; form into patties and fry. Quick and good!

Red Snapper in Tomato Sauce

red snapper	1 tablespoon flour
salt substitute	½ cup butter
1 chopped onion	2 tablespoons chopped celery
1 chopped green pepper	1 clove garlic
2 bay leaves	1 can tomato soup
Worcestershire sauce	1 tablespoon ketchup

Sprinkle flour on fish. In a separate pan simmer in butter the onions, celery and pepper until these ingredients are tender. Then add the tomato soup and the other ingredients. Pour over fish and bake at 350° for about an hour. Baste with the sauce during the baking.

Baked Fish

For this dish you may use striped bass, red snapper, carp, mackerel or almost any other fish.

1 small striped bass	paprika
1 onion	1 lemon
salt substitute	1 can tomatoes
1 clove garlic	vegetable oil
parsley	

Slice the onion and sauté in oil until golden brown, then add tomatoes, garlic, paprika, salt substitute and lemon juice. Cook for about half an hour. Place fish in baking dish and cover with sauce. Bake at 400° for half an hour. Garnish with chopped parsley and onion wedges.

Broiled Fish

When broiling any of the fish mentioned in these recipes or menus we recommend that you not dredge the slices in flour; a sprinkling of flour may be all right, but don't go beyond that. You may brush the slices with a small amount of vegetable oil and you should make sure that the broiling rack is so coated. This will, of course, prevent the fish from sticking when you go to turn it. Remember that fish is naturally tender; you cook it to provide more flavor—that is the reason you use certain ingredients in the cooking. Do not overcook. Most fish will cook in five to ten minutes. It is always a good idea to baste the fish in its own juice.

Allowable Salads

Lobster Salad

fresh lobster chunks
house dressing
chopped green pepper
sherry

chopped or grated onion
chopped celery
radishes

Mix the above ingredients together until they assume as close to a homogenous consistency as possible. Serve on a couple of lettuce leaves. Check back in this book to review the ingredients for the house dressing. CAUTION: No more than one tablespoon of wine per salad, and no bread or crackers with it.

Chicken Salad

A good thing to keep in mind about chicken salad (or turkey, or duck or veal salad) is that the finished dish should still taste of its main ingredient. So don't overwhelm it with vegetables and seasonings and dressings. We want you to get mostly protein, not carbohydrate. A good rule of thumb in making any salad (and we will be having more of them on Day 7) is to keep the main ingredient proportionately three times greater than anything else in the mixture. That way you will still be able to tell what *kind* of salad it is, but you will also get the subsidiary subtle flavorings and crunchiness.

To make an unroutine chicken salad, try the following:

cooked chicken sliced into
    small, bite-sized pieces
1 chopped onion
1 chopped green pepper
1 tablespoon chopped celery

lettuce leaves
chopped stuffed olives
lemon juice
house dressing

After mixing together the basic ingredients, add salad dressing to proper consistency (not too loose) and flavor with pepper and salt substitute, or just a pinch of regular salt. Sprinkle with paprika and a small amount of chopped parsley, or use several sprigs of parsley to dress up the plate.

A FEW BRIEF REMINDERS

1. Remember that when cooking fowl, you will be able to eat the skin. In fact, we usually tell patients that we don't care if they eat the right side of the chicken, the left side, the skin, the feet and the neck. We also suggest that you eat the giblets, which are delicious fried separately in a Teflon pan and served with the roasted bird. So it is fine with us if you flavor the skin. We suggest that you cook it so that it becomes crisp; you shouldn't eat it fatty. Remember, these meals of yours are meant to be pleasant as well as filling. That's why we've taken a lot of time selecting menu alternatives for you. Take advantage of our research—and your own cooking skills.

2. Don't make up your own recipes, attempting to substitute something you like for something you don't care for as much. Even if you think the calories are the same, chances are they are not. Even if the caloric value *is* similar, what you select may interfere with some other item for the day of our selection. All we will be doing, then, is fighting one another, and we don't want to fight with you. Don't forget, going off our Plan means going back on your own—and remember what yours did to you.

3. Where recipes call for using vegetables that may not appear on your own menu, don't eat them. Serve them to the others at the table. If your menu calls for other vegetables, stick to those. That doesn't mean you have to be "different" from everyone else at the table; for children, especially, this is a hardship. You can share your vegetables with everyone else. Pass them around, but just don't feel obligated to try others that do not apply to you.

4. You will note that neither here nor in the previous chapter have we spent time dealing with food that is NOT permitted. We feel there is no necessity for this, because if you don't find it on your menu sections, as far as you are concerned it doesn't exist—at least for that day. There are a number of reasons why certain foods are here and others aren't. It doesn't mean that those items we have left out of the Plan aren't nutritious, wholesome foods; it merely means that we have found them difficult to utilize for a rapid CBO—and that is what we are all interested in, isn't it?

5. Finally, we want to say a word about measurements. You should weigh all the items that call for weighing, at least initially.

194

You will quickly learn to distinguish between four- or six- or eight-ounce items, but don't assume that you can do so without weighing at first. Your eye will deceive you. Invest in a small, inexpensive postal scale. Many items, of course (such as meats), provide an indication of weight on the package, making it easy for you to subdivide it to your requirements. Do this as soon as you get home; wrap each "ration" and freeze it against the time of its use. This will establish a useful pattern that will put the correct portions of food right in your hand at the time you require them.

Here are some weight and measure equivalents you might find useful:

6 teaspoons = 1 ounce
3 teaspoons = 1 tablespoon
1 cup = 8 ounces
1 pint = 1 pound

Remember, it is important that, whatever you are eating, you eat it slowly. Chew well; chew liquids as well as solids to slow down your eating time. Learn to make the most of the very least; that way you will find yourself making more of it. A good example may be drawn from the measurements above. You can see that it takes six teaspoonfuls to make one ounce. The average forkful should be approximately one teaspoonful. One ounce of food, therefore, would be six forkfuls. If you take your time, chew each forkful of food with care, put your fork back on the table during this process and drink water between bites, you can make your single ounce of food last quite a while. Of course, we are not limiting you to a single ounce of food to eat. But if it takes three minutes to eat six bites (one ounce), and the average meal consists of ten to fifteen ounces, you should be able to sit at the table for at least half an hour—which is longer than most families do sit for a meal despite all the talk of "togetherness" at mealtimes. You will feel a lot more satisfied eating this way than you did when you were gulping down a mountain of food and feeling hungry again in a couple of hours. Better yet, eating according to your Nine-Day menus and taking it a bite at a time, chewing well, will begin to dissolve all the weight you have accumulated by trying to diet it off on other plans. Here you will not only be satisfied by what you are taking in, but by what you are taking off. Not only will you see and feel a miraculous difference, but everyone will start telling you how great you look—like a totally different person. And you will know it is true because that is precisely what you will have become.

10 FRIDAY: THE VEGETABLE, FRUIT AND DAIRY DAY

You are now approaching the end of the five-day midweek sector and you have every right to feel darn good about things. Tomorrow you will be weighing yourself for the second time, and if you have been following the Plan carefully you can look forward to a substantial weight loss. You should feel good not only mentally, realizing that you have been controlling a situation that has managed to slip out of your grasp on past occasions, but physically as well.

"I don't know what it is about your Plan," a patient recently confessed, "but I go back on it quite often even though I'm now at my ideal weight. It's not that I want to lose more weight, but I find I have more energy when I'm on the Wonder Diet, I sleep more soundly—and I require less sleep. Yet I feel sharper during the day."

We hear that all the time. In fact, we ourselves go back on the Plan on occasion even though we are both now at normal weight. We find it a wonderful source of physical energy and a way of relaxing the body's mental knots as well. Why is this? Well, the energy saved by not being wasted on digestion of surplus food, plus the energy potential of the foods recommended in the particular

197

sequences, *plus* the energy released by the burning of accumulated fat make a pretty good metabolic package that should not only sail you through the normal activities of your day, but give you plenty of zip for after-work activities. At the same time, the precise discipline of each day's diet takes the anxiety off your shoulders about planning your meals in a way that will make you a healthier human being. So why shouldn't you feel better all around—and look better as well?

IT'S YOUR OBLIGATION TO KEEP YOUNG

If you're a fat woman, aren't you fed up with hearing people say: "She's got such a pretty face." Or, if you are a fat man, "He could be so good-looking."—as though physical beauty were the be-all and end-all of existence and all we have going for us is attractiveness! Yet none of us can deny that we enjoy being complimented. It is a fact of life that physical attractiveness is a major source of compliments, whether spoken or implied. And looking and keeping young adds immeasurably to our attractiveness regardless of our actual age, regardless of how plain our features may be. We believe that everyone has a duty to keep as young as possible for as long as possible. Losing only twenty pounds will make you, quite literally, younger.Even at this point in the Nine-Day Plan, you are probably looking...and feeling...younger than you have in years. You will see the change yourself in your next picture. We are used to seeing it in our office patients. A common remark by them is: "Doctor, you've taken years off my age." What we've really done is worked with Nature to give you another chance at years that were wasted. We've told you before that there are no miracles in dieting, that it is all hard, precise work. Yet isn't this a miracle of sorts? To be almost able to go back in time, to be younger? Part of the reason for this effect is the foods we have selected for the Nine-Day Plan: all natural, wholesome foods, to be prepared in ways that will preserve the basic nutrition that Nature has stored within them. We have always found that working with Nature is 90 percent of any battle in medicine; it is no different in the Battle of the Bulge. Nature is the best physician of all; she was in practice long before physicians were invented.

198

SPEAKING OF NATURAL FOODS

Today's diet will give you a good idea of how many vegetarians get by, yet it is not really a vegetarian diet; at least we don't like to think of it that way and would prefer you not to. It is merely one more link in the chain of your mounting weight loss, all of which will be accumulated at the end of the Nine-Day Cycle. Today you will be eating foods practically out of Nature's laboratory; for many of you these meals should be a real treat, especially if you've convinced yourself over the years that you're not a meat or fish eater. And you will be surprised at how well satisfied you can be with these foods even if over the years you've convinced yourself that all you are *is* a meat or fish eater.

"But," one of our patients said in dismay, "aren't these foods mostly carbohydrates? Aren't they full of calories... and won't they make me fatter?" The answer to that, of course, is, "Not at all." Not if you eat them according to the way we have arranged them for you. Not if you eat according to past instructions. In fact, you will find that you can get quite comfortably full on these foods as we provide them and, because of their fibrous nature, stay full and comfortable for quite a long time. The first thing you must do is to think of them as foods—not merely as adjuncts to the dinner plate; not merely as excuses to take a piece of bread or a lot of salt or to quench your thirst; not as snacks. As with all your other foods, you will sit down to eat these; you will pay attention only to them—not to a book or TV—treating them with the respect due important objects; you will chew slowly and put the fruit or the fork down between bites. That's the natural way to eat.

WHAT YOU WILL EAT TODAY

1. Eight glasses of cold water divided over the day. By this time you should be getting pretty good at water drinking. Did you find it difficult when you began? Wasn't that silly? Look how you have improved in just this aspect alone. It is, we hope, going to be a habit that you will carry with you all your life. Together with your weight loss, it may just make your life last longer.

2. Your multi-vitamin-mineral tablet or tablets if you are taking more than one. We have had patients who felt that they would need extra vitamins as they "always got sick" on diets. Well, we have never had a patient we were treating personally get sick on our diet, but if you feel that extra vitamins will help see you through the Plan, it is a small enough price to pay for success.

3. Your "total contentment" pill (if you so desire).

4. Tea or coffee may be taken at will throughout the day. For today you may take up to three teaspoons of whole milk in your coffee or tea provided you do not drink more than five cups for the day. If you will be drinking more than that, switch to one teaspoon of nondairy creamer.

5. You may have the following fruit snacks between meals today: half a grapefruit, one medium pear, one medium plum, one medium guava, one medium orange or nectarine. It is NOT ESSENTIAL that you eat these. You may, if you wish, select any two of the above as snacks, but no more than that. We suggest that you save one of the two selected snack fruits for sometime after dinner. Do not eat *anything* later than two hours before going to bed at night.

6. You may have up to three cans of diet soda today. Remember, you may not substitute this for your water; nor does the coffee or tea you drink substitute for your water.

The times for your eating are, as usual, very specific. They are the same times we have been using through the week (refer back to Chapter 9). And (we hate to keep repeating this, but our office patients continually come in with the complaint "I can't eat all that food."): *You don't have to eat everything on the menu.* You can eat less. Just don't eat more. No substituting or saving calories from one meal to the next.

PREPARING TODAY'S FOOD

Preparation for today will be highly specific, with each dish having its preparation indicated where we feel this is necessary. (Consult the Recipe section.) We have tried to make all the menus as tasty and as appetizing as possible while sticking to preparations that do not require a gourmet education. The idea here is to lose weight, but also to make the experience as pleasant as possible. It amuses us to find how many of our patients find it initially so difficult to cope with weight loss as a pleasant experience. They are used to the old adage about medicine: The more unpleasant it is, the better it works. "I feel sinful having such a good time eating and losing weight as well," one patient told us the other day. But that's the way it is on the Nine-Day Plan; you might as well get used to it.

BASIC MENU: DAY 7

Breakfast *4 oz. tomato juice*
2 eggs: do them differently; if frying, use a Teflon pan.
2 pieces Melba toast
4 oz. skim milk or buttermilk
coffee, tea

Lunch *4 oz. honeydew melon*
8 oz. Special Nine-Day Fruit Salad
4 oz. skim milk
coffee, tea

Dinner *8 oz. Friday Salad*
8 oz. Special Nine-Day Casserole
2 pieces Melba toast
4 oz. skim milk
coffee, tea

For all dishes whose ingredients are not specifically noted, look in the Recipe section. We think you will be pleasantly surprised to find how much variety you are able to eat—yet how few calories you will be taking in. We have spent a good bit of time on these recipes, have tried all of them ourselves and can testify to their efficacy as both culinary treats and weight-loss aids. For even further variations on today's food, the following alternatives are at your (quite literal) service:

Alternate Menu #1: Combining Vegetables, Fruit, Dairy

Breakfast *4 oz. orange juice*
2 pieces Melba toast
8 oz. skim milk

Lunch *⅓ cup cottage cheese*
½ cup peaches
½ cup pears

½ cup celery
4 oz. lettuce
4 oz. green pepper
½ cup skim milk or buttermilk
coffee, tea

Dinner 4 oz. tomato juice
Special Dish: Fried Eggplant with Cheese
½ cup cantaloupe balls
coffee, tea

Alternate Menu #2: Combining Vegetables, Fruit, Dairy

Breakfast 1 orange (medium)
1 egg, boiled or poached (use salt substitute or pepper)
1 piece Melba toast
½ cup whole milk
coffee, tea

Lunch 2-inch wedge honeydew melon
6 stalks of fresh or canned asparagus
½ cup chopped onion
½ cup green peppers
4 oz. tomatoes
4 oz. raw spinach
½ cup raw carrot
Dressing: vinegar, lemon juice or house dressing
½ cup whole milk
coffee, tea

Dinner ½ cup Campbell's split pea soup
Special Nine-Day Baked Zucchini Dish
4 oz. unflavored yogurt
coffee, tea

Alternate Menu #3: Combining Vegetables and Fruit

Breakfast 4 oz. tomato juice
8 oz. fruit cup consisting of slices of grapefruit, orange, cantaloupe, strawberries, 2 oz. yogurt
coffee, tea

Lunch *6 oz. V-8 juice*
8 oz. total of vegetable salad consisting of: lima beans, macaroni, tomatoes, celery, green pepper. Flavor with vinegar, lemon juice or house dressing
3 oz. unflavored yogurt
coffee, tea
Dinner *4 oz. Campbell's black bean soup*
8 oz. Special Eggplant Soufflé
coffee, tea

Alternate Menu #4: Combining Vegetables and Fruit

Breakfast *4 oz. apple juice (bottled or canned)*
8 oz. Orange-Ginger Surprise
coffee, tea
Lunch *6 oz. Campbell's Chunky Vegetable soup*
Special Chick-Pea Salad
coffee, tea
Dinner *4 oz. tomato cocktail*
8 oz. vegetable fritters
2 oz. unflavored yogurt
coffee, tea

Alternate Menu #5: Combining Vegetables and Dairy

Breakfast *½ cup V-8 juice*
2 eggs, fried (use Teflon), poached or hard-boiled
1 piece Melba toast
coffee, tea
Lunch *1 cup borscht*
1 medium potato
2 tablespoons sour cream
coffee, tea
Dinner *4 oz. tomato juice*
8 oz. cheese pancakes
1 cup skim milk
coffee, tea

203

Alternate Menu #6: Combining Vegetables and Dairy

Breakfast *1 cup Kellogg's cornflakes*
8 oz. whole milk (no more than 1 percent fat)
2 pieces Melba toast
1 teaspoon Smucker's jelly
coffee, tea

Lunch *4 oz. tomato or V-8 juice*
4 oz. Lipton or Campbell's vegetable soup (or homemade vegetable soup)*
8 oz. Special Caesar Salad
1 cup skim milk
coffee, tea

Dinner *4 oz. celery stuffed with ⅓ cup creamed cottage cheese or pot cheese*
1 piece Ry-Krisp
1 egg, fried (use Teflon), poached or hard-boiled
coffee, tea

*Both Campbell's and Heinz make a canned (prepared with water, according to directions on container) vegetarian soup that may be substituted here.

Alternate Menu #7: Combining Fruit and Dairy

Breakfast *½ grapefruit*
1 soft, hard-boiled or poached egg
1 piece Melba toast
1 teaspoon jelly
coffee, tea

Lunch *8-oz. fruit cup consisting of watermelon, honeydew, orange and grapefruit slices, pineapple, strawberries*
⅓ cup cottage cheese
1 cup skim milk
coffee, tea

Dinner *4 oz. grapes*
8 oz. Special Apple Salad
1 cup skim milk or buttermilk

coffee, tea

Alternate Menu #8: Combining Fruit and Dairy

Breakfast *1 orange*
1 cup regular Cream of Wheat
½ cup whole milk
coffee, tea

Lunch *4 oz. strawberries*
½ cup skim milk
6 oz. Special Pear and Cheese Dish

Dinner *4 oz. applesauce*
1 egg (omelet)
1 piece Melba toast
coffee, tea

Alternate Menu #9: Vegetables Alone

Breakfast *4 oz. tomato juice*
1 slice banana bread
coffee, tea

Lunch *8 oz. mushroom soup*
8 oz. Special Spinach Salad
2 pieces Ry-Krisp
coffee, tea

Dinner *4 oz. V-8 juice*
8 oz. Special Broccoli-Cauliflower Compote
4 oz. raw carrot and celery sticks
3 oz. unflavored yogurt
coffee, tea

Alternate Menu #10: Vegetables Alone

Breakfast *4 oz. V-8 juice*
2 pieces Melba toast
1 teaspoon jelly
coffee, tea

Lunch *4 oz. raw celery and carrot sticks*
8 oz. Special Grilled Tomato Dish
coffee, tea

Dinner *8 oz. lettuce and tomato salad with lemon juice dressing*
2 regular slices toasted bread: white, whole-wheat or rye,
with 8 stalks asparagus tips (fresh or canned) as open
sandwich
½ cup canned corn or 1 small ear of fresh corn
coffee, tea

Alternate Menu #11: Fruit Alone
Breakfast *1 orange*
2 pieces Ry-Krisp
1 tablespoon any fruit jelly or preserve
coffee, tea
Lunch *8 oz. Special Nine-Day Fruit Bowl*
1 slice bread (regular)
coffee, tea
Dinner *½ grapefruit*
8 oz. Special Cherry-Banana Salad
coffee, tea

Alternate Menu #12: Fruit Alone
Breakfast *½ grapefruit*
1 blueberry muffin
1 teaspoon any jelly (fruit) or preserve
coffee, tea
Lunch *4 oz. dish of strawberries*
1 slice banana-nut bread
4 oz. any fruit-flavored yogurt
coffee, tea
Dinner *4 oz. stewed prunes*
1 slice cinnamon-raisin bread
coffee, tea

Alternate Menu #13: Dairy Alone
Breakfast *⅔ cup corn flakes*
½ cup whole milk
1 slice thin bread
1 teaspoon butter
coffee, tea

Lunch *8 oz. skim milk or buttermilk*
cheese omelet consisting of one egg, no more than 1 oz.
cheese
coffee, tea

Dinner *8 oz. plain yogurt*
coffee, tea

In the above menu, lunch and dinner may be exchanged depending on which time you feel hungriest.

Alternate Menu #14: Dairy Alone

Breakfast *1 glass (8 oz.) whole milk*
1 slice thin toast
1 teaspoon jelly
coffee, tea

Lunch *1 large biscuit shredded wheat*
                    OR
¼ cup grapenuts
1 glass skim milk
2 pieces Melba toast
coffee, tea

Dinner *8-oz. glass skim milk or buttermilk*
1-egg omelet that may be combined with 3 asparagus stalks, ¼ cup chopped onion, ¼ cup chopped green pepper (see Recipe section)
1 piece Melba toast
coffee, tea

SOMETHING FOR EVERYONE

Now, it may appear that we have presented you with a great selection of choices for a single day's dieting, as indeed we have done in the past chapters. However, we have found that when dealing with specific foods and specific amounts, as one must do in the Nine-Day Plan, there must be something for everyone, and this we have attempted to provide. But there is another reason for the carefully chosen alternate menus. You will see, at the end of the book, that we will be using these menus as part of the Cycle Balancing Plan that will guide you from the end of one Cycle to the beginning of the next—assuming, of course, that you have more weight to lose than can be handled comfortably by a single cycle of the Nine-Day Wonder Diet. In addition, they will form a number of interesting variations from the original base plan that may be used to speed up or level out weight loss depending on *your* assessment of the situation. And, finally, we will combine these alternate menus into still different groupings when we discuss rapid weight loss with regard to food allergies, illnesses, the specific ways to diet at work, home and at school, and the best combinations for various age groupings. So you see, everything in this book is important in one way or another; if we are talking in the main to 90 percent of our readers, we still want to take the effort to provide a workable plan for the remaining 10 percent as well. In point of fact we are really talking to a single individual: YOU! You are the one we must reach; you are the one who has probably tried everything else by now and found that what may have looked good for you, initially, in the long run turned out to be developed for someone else. The Nine-Day Wonder Diet is YOUR plan. We have done our best to tailor it to your needs and comforts. Once you try it on for size, you'll find that you will fit into it more rapidly than you ever thought possible—and it won't be the Plan that will be doing the shrinking.

RECIPES FOR DAY 7
Special Nine-Day Fruit Bowl (Salad)
Cut a large watermelon about a quarter down from the top; take the top section off. With a scoop remove most of the watermelon pulp. This will serve as your salad bowl; if you don't want to get fancy just employ a standard salad bowl. Mix two tablespoons fresh lemon juice, anise seed and salt substitute in a cup of water and cook it to a syrupy state. Chill immediately. Cut up a pineapple, cantaloupe, watermelon, apple, pear and oranges into bite-size pieces; add grapes and slices of peaches and plums. Pour over this mixture the chilled syrup from the refrigerator.

Fried Eggplant With Cheese

olive oil	*garlic*
onion	*canned tomatoes*
about ½ cup flour	*1 egg, beaten*
eggplant, sliced	*Parmesan cheese*
Feta cheese	*pepper*

208

Sauté some chopped garlic with oil, add onions and tomatoes and let simmer for thirty minutes. Prepare a batter by mixing flour and egg. Dip eggplant slices in batter and fry until light brown. Preheat oven to 350° and place slices of eggplant in pan with sauce between layers and pieces of Feta cheese. Sprinkle each layer with Parmesan cheese. Bake until cheese melts. If you wish, you may add sliced olives, stuffed with pimento, between layers.

Special Nine-Day Zucchini Dish

5 medium zucchini	garlic
parsley	butter
salt substitute	Lawry's seasoned pepper
Feta cheese	grated Parmesan cheese

Zucchini should be cut lengthwise and put into baking dish that has been greased with butter. Mix together garlic, parsley and butter, and place a dollop on each long zucchini slice. Now sprinkle the Feta cheese and Parmesan on each slice. Put directly under broiler for five to seven minutes. Test for zucchini's tenderness with fork.

Eggplant Soufflé

¼ cup butter	six egg yolks and whites, separated
1 cup skimmed milk	
¼ cup Parmesan cheese	Feta cheese
2 eggplants	cinnamon to taste
2 tablespoons flour	

Take the pulp from the eggplant and chop finely. Melt butter in double boiler, adding flour slowly. Add milk and stir, then add egg yolks and the two cheeses slowly, after removing the inner pot from the water; you may have to put the pot back in the water to get the cheese to melt. Add seasonings. When mixture is quite cool, mix in the eggplant pulp. Then mix in the egg whites (beaten until stiff). Place in soufflé dish in oven; cook until brown.

Orange-Ginger Surprise

orange sections	diet ginger ale
finely chopped fresh mint	

Prepare the orange slices from seedless oranges if possible, or from nectarines. Place the slices in glasses, add diet ginger ale and sprinkle mint over the top. You may use the whole mint leaf if it is fresh.

Chick-Pea Salad

1 can chick-peas	salt substitute
1 teaspoon lemon juice	olive oil
unsalted peanuts	garlic
bay leaf	parsley

Purée the chick-peas by mashing them with a fork. Add a half cup water and lemon juice and mix until thoroughly blended. Crush the peanuts and add small amount of olive oil until the mix is a paste. Add this to the lemon-water mix; add garlic, salt substitute and crushed bay leaf. Serve chilled, garnished with parsley.

Vegetable Fritters

cauliflower	zucchini
eggplant	potato
parsnips	squash
flour	lemon juice
salt substitute	pepper
olives	olive oil

Boil all the vegetables until tender (peel potatoes). Cut into slices when cool. Mix flour, lemon juice, seasoning, chopped olives (and pimentos) and olive oil. You may add a dash of white wine. Heat olive oil in pan, dip vegetable slices in batter and fry until brown. Drain oil before eating.

Cheese Pancakes

2 egg whites	1 cup flour
1 cup skim milk	1 teaspoon baking powder
salt substitute	olive oil
pot cheese (not creamed)	

Mix flour, salt substitute, baking powder. Add this mix to the egg whites, along with the milk, cheese and a small amount of oil. Heat oil in large skillet. When hot, place the batter, a tablespoonful at a time, into the oil. Brown on both sides, turning with care. DRAIN OIL WELL BEFORE EATING.

Caesar Salad

olive oil	lemon juice
garlic (crushed)	salt substitute
pepper	lettuce
croutons	Feta cheese
sardines	hard-boiled egg
olives (stuffed with pimentos)	celery stalks
carrot	green pepper

Cut all ingredients to bite size, mix well in large bowl. Add olive oil, lemon juice, salt substitute and pepper to taste. Variation: You may use raw egg rather than hard-boiled, and anchovies rather than sardines.

Apple Salad

apples	cottage cheese
pears	yogurt
lemon juice	cinnamon
grapes	dry sherry

Mix above ingredients (fruit should be cut to bite-size pieces) and blend well with cottage cheese. Add yogurt to thin the mix, cinnamon to taste. Should be served chilled. Add sherry only before serving.

Pear and Cheese Dish

6 pears	¼ cup diet sweetener
lemon juice	margarine
Brie or Camembert cheese	

Use fresh pears only; peel but do not core or slice them. Heat diet sweetener, lemon juice and margarine in a cup of water until it boils. Place pears in oven dish, add lemon mix from stove. Bake at 325°, covered, for about one hour. Place in refrigerator when done; serve by slicing pears and placing slices of cheese on top.

Spinach Salad

sesame seed	salad oil
soy sauce	Worcestershire sauce
hot pepper	spinach leaves, raw
salt substitute	pepper
carrot slices	garlic powder

Mix and stir well the sesame seed, salad oil, soy sauce and a dash of Worcestershire. Add remainder of ingredients after tearing spinach leaves to roughly bite-size pieces. Flavor with condiments to taste. Serve chilled after tossing.

Broccoli-Cauliflower Dish

broccoli	olives (you may use green stuffed with pimento)
olive oil	
Parmesan cheese	Feta cheese
garlic	salt substitute
cauliflower	

Cook broccoli and cauliflower in boiling water until tender. Heat oil with garlic slices, then remove garlic. Place vegetables, sliced, in hot oil; season while they simmer. Add olives, sliced. Remove from pan, sprinkle with Parmesan cheese, garnish with Feta.

Grilled Tomatoes

tomatoes (ripe ones, please)	chopped onion
chopped carrots	chopped celery
chopped green pepper	bread crumbs
salt substitute	Lawry's Seasoned Pepper
Feta cheese	grated cheddar cheese
olive oil	

After cutting the tops off the tomatoes, scoop out the pulp. Do not go near the skin. Mix together onion, celery, green pepper, carrots, tomato pulp and Feta cheese. Add bread crumbs to the olive oil and mix that in. Fill each tomato shell with the mix, and bake for about one hour. Before serving, remove from oven, sprinkle with cheddar cheese and return to oven until cheese melts.

212

Cherry-Banana Salad

sour cream   *sweet or sour cherries*
bananas   *diet sweetener*

Mix the sour cream and the diet sweetener; you may add a little cinnamon. Mix in cherries and bananas. EAT SLOWLY.

Broiled Grapefruit

It is a good idea to keep in mind that this fruit, so flexible in its use on the Nine-Day Plan, may be eaten cooked as well as raw. It is quite delicious this way. Cut the grapefruit and remove as many seeds as possible. Sprinkle with a little diet sweetener, broil for about ten minutes. Serve garnished with parsley or fresh mint. It is a meal in itself.

Omelets

Where indicated, eggs may be made into "containing" omelets. For these, the most common additions are onion, mushroom, pepper (green) and asparagus. Wherever a choice of eggs is allowed, you may make an omelet containing not more than ½ cup of the above. (You may, of course, eat the omelet plain if you prefer.)

LOOKING FORWARD AND BACKWARD

You have now completed an entire week on the Nine-Day Plan. You are almost home-free—free of a good deal, if not all, of that excessive weight that has plagued you for so long.

Can you believe you've gotten this far so easily? "I can't believe I've almost done it," patients usually marvel at the point. And then they add, "You know, I was eating fine until the fast days; now I just can't seem to take in all the food that is allowed."

Well, that's fine. We don't object to this change in your eating. Nor should you. Remember what we keep telling you: The Nine-Day Plan is quite flexible. You must find within it those applications that best suit *you.* The fact that we have built into the basic structure certain options applicable to someone who "eats like a horse" doesn't mean that *you* have to eat like one just because the food may be "allowed." Better to speak like a horse and say: "Nay."

But if you think that you are eating more just because it is on the menu, and not because you are truly hungry, don't worry about it.

213

Finish the cycle. You'll still have lost weight. And next time around, try one of the rapid-loss variations in the next-to-last chapter. It may be that the cycle food is so tempting from the standpoint of sheer variety that your appetite is stimulated and you are eating more than your hunger calls for on this basis alone. Again, finish the cycle and then, if you still have weight to lose, try the specific "monotony cycle" in the next-to-last chapter. This may be the variation just calculated to your needs. The same chapter will be of help if you have been feeling frustrated because you are really a "nibbler" and provision hasn't been made for the way you really feel is the best way for you to eat on the basic Plan. Continual munching can still take pounds off you and, in this variation, eating times are done away with.

The main point is this: As you now approach the final stage in your first cycle, don't have any doubts about your eventual success. To change long-standing eating habits abruptly is far from easy for most people. This may have caused you to cheat a bit here and there as you went along on your first nine days. It's only human; let us work with you a little more fully next time. But never, never quit in the middle of a cycle. Remember, we've allowed for your falterings—and that's all they are, not stumbling blocks. If this first cycle has brought out any hesitations in your progress, that's a good, not a bad thing. Now you know what little inconsistencies have to be rectified. Chances are that you will find, in the next-to-last chapter, that we've already taken care of them.

So we repeat: For no reason should you pause now, on the very threshold of ultimate success. Finish the cycle, even if you think you've done badly by not following directions. Next time will be easier and, if necessary, you can incorporate some of the unique variations from the last chapter to make it easier still.

So much for the small percentage of you who may have had uncertainties. For the rest of you, by far the majority as our experience has shown, you probably don't need or want any modifications. Your needs have been met. Your weight has been lost, with more to go. But don't let yourself be carried away by success. Finish up with a good sprint on the weekend. The race you are running is one toward your goal of ideal weight and slimness. You've never been closer to it than you are at this minute.

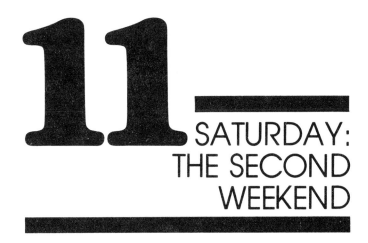

SATURDAY: THE SECOND WEEKEND

The first thing you are going to do today is weigh yourself. Follow the instructions for your previous weighing, keeping in mind that you still have two days to go on the Plan. Whether you have lost more than you anticipated or less, *you must finish out the cycle.* Believe it or not, more people seem to fall off the Plan at this critical juncture than at any other time during the nine days. One woman reported that she was very disheartened because she'd lost only five pounds by this second Saturday. She was ready to cry; we could hear the tears in her voice over the telephone.

Fortunately, we were able to convince her to stay with the Plan over the second weekend. She was dubious, but promised to do so. Her reward—and ours—was the jubilant phone call we got on Monday reporting an additional four pounds lost over the weekend. Nevertheless she was puzzled. "I can't understand how I lost four pounds in one weekend and only five during the previous seven days," she said.

Well, the reason is simple. As we explained to her, she really hadn't lost the four additional pounds based on what she had done on the second weekend alone. The loss of those four pounds was really due as much to everything she'd done *up to* that second weekend as to what she'd done *on* it. By staying on the Plan right

215

up to the end she had permitted her accumulated fat mobilization to peak and the excess fat so gathered to be oxidized (burned) by her normal body processes. That is why the Nine-Day Plan takes nine days, not seven or eight.

Let's just take a moment to examine this a little more closely. What you have accomplished so far, though it has taken most of the cycle, is really only half the battle. What you have accomplished so far is not only weight loss but, more important, the potential for further weight loss. Unfortunately, it is only weight loss that shows on the scale; there is no way for you to measure weight-loss potential. Take our word for it, however, as did the woman on the phone, that this is a very real force, one that can either make everything you have done so far into a success, or let you turn it into a failure. And, as we pointed out, that goes for those of you who may, right now, be more than satisfied with the amount of weight you've already lost. You may be saying to yourself: "I've done really well up to this point; I don't need to lose any more. Why bother to continue?" Well, we'd like to point out that one reason for continuing is that you can't have too much of a good thing; but another, and more pressing, reason is that if you stop now you, like the individual who may think he hasn't lost enough, will be backsliding. You will be wasting a good portion of the time and effort of the past week. You will not lose all the weight that your efforts have deserved—and, even more tragic, you are liable to gain back pounds you lost just by not completing the cycle for the two days that remain. Is it worth it? Certainly not. Remember, the game is never over until the last inning is played. These last two days are critical; don't slough them off.

YOUR CALORIE BURN-OUT CONTINUES

There is still one more reason for finishing the nine days of the cycle, regardless of what your weight may be this morning. And it is this. We know that just as a skier on a hill generates momentum as he descends—momentum that can take him with ease over the next hill (provided he doesn't fall over)—your Calory Burn-Out, invested with the momentum of the past nine days, will continue to work for you even after your cycle is over. We discovered this quite

216

by accident. A number of our patients, carried away by the weight they had lost during their Nine-Day Diet, immediately went back to eating pretty much according to their "normal" pattern. That is to say, they gorged themselves—this despite our specific instructions to the contrary. *And yet they continued to lose weight.* Amazing, isn't it? Of course, eventually they found that their weight loss began to level off and, when they persisted in eating the wrong foods in inordinate amounts, they began gaining weight again. Yet for a while they were able to coast just on the momentum they had built up during the time they had spent on the Plan. It follows that the more time on the Plan you allow yourself, the more coasting you can do afterward, the more time you will have to accustom yourself to proper eating: healthful and comfortable eating, without the specter of overweight arising to challenge you. That's why we urge you to start your Nine-Day Plan NOW. Don't wait until that wedding or anniversary that's coming up is over to start dieting. Don't say to yourself, "As soon as my vacation is over, I'll start to lose weight." If you start *before* these events are due, you can lose your weight and still keep it off by virtue of the *potential* weight loss you still have coming. No one objects to a bonus. Here's one you can supply yourself with. Stick with the Plan right to the end: cash in instead of checking out. You'll be glad you did.

WHAT YOU WILL EAT TODAY

1. Eight glasses of cold water spread throughout the day.

2. Your multivitamin-mineral tablet.

3. Your "total contentment" pill (again, this is your choice).

4. Tea and/or coffee. Today you must drink your coffee black. Tea is to be taken only with lemon, no milk. You may use artificial sweetener.

5. Choose from the following fruits to be eaten three times during the day, not less than three hours apart. You may choose the same fruit three times if you like, or you may vary them. Do not exceed the amounts given:

4 oz. cranberries
4 oz. strawberries
1 wedge honeydew melon

4 oz. watermelon
½ medium cantaloupe.
When eating the above, try to eat as slowly as possible. Sit down. Give your jaws "chewing time." We have purposely picked items that must go on a plate; that way you will be reminded to sit at the table to eat. You may use the fruits as snacks between meals or as a snack prior to bedtime. Do not eat anything within one hour of retiring for the night.

6. You may have up to two cans of diet soda today.

Eating times are the same as they have been through the week. The Basic Menu for today is provided below; as usual, alternate menus will follow. Please remember that if you dislike a certain food, or if you are allergic to certain items, we do not want you to eat them. We have, throughout the Plan, given you enough choice to be able to have you work around any foods you may find objectionable for any reason.

Remember: Dieting on the Nine-Day Wonder Diet is not meant to be a punishment; it is meant to be a relief from punishment. You've already punished yourself quite enough the way you've been eating. On the Nine-Day Plan you can relax, eat and lose weight without worrying. The built-in willpower in the Plan will do all your worrying for you. Isn't that nice?

BASIC MENU: DAY 8

Breakfast 1 orange
1 egg, boiled or poached
1 piece Ry-Krisp
coffee, tea

Lunch ⅓ cup cottage cheese
4 oz. lettuce
4 oz. cucumber
6 stalks asparagus
2 slices tomato
1 piece Ry-Krisp
coffee, tea

Dinner 4 oz. chicken (breast only)
4 oz. cauliflower

218

4 oz. string beans
4 oz. beets (fresh or canned)
4 oz. lettuce
coffee, tea
Snack before bedtime: ½ cup skim milk.

SATURDAY VARIATIONS
If You Are a Dating Single

Most diets are based on a strict formula. In these plans all overweights are considered strictly fat problems and rules are laid down that apply strictly to fat. However, as we keep pointing out, individual considerations are what really make any diet plan successful. Your Nine-Day Wonder Diet is an individual plan tailored to your specific needs.

We recognize, for instance, that for the single, dating overweight male or female Saturday night can pose very special problems. This is especially true of the second Saturday in the cycle in which, quite frankly, the food intake has been considerably cut down from what it was on the first weekend. Now, if you are a dating single, rest assured that our years of experience spent counseling people with weight problems have taught us the most efficient method of guiding *you*. Your problems are not unique. And it's from our experience with problems like yours that we know enough not to ask you (as so many diets do) to stay home and "avoid temptation." The Nine-Day Wonder Diet is not a punishment. We want you to go out and enjoy yourself. All we ask is that you be prepared—emotionally as well as dietarily. The following "action line" will help put you in the best possible shape for your evening out. In this way you will have nothing to reproach yourself for when you return home.

1. Admit to yourself that you are fat and that your extra poundage will be coming along for the evening. Your weight isn't something you can subdivide, leaving a portion back home and temporarily forgetting about it. We all like to have a good time and pack our troubles away. However, *your* good time can be extended, not abbreviated, by keeping your goal of slimness in mind.

2. Do your best to disguise your weight comfortably. It is fine to

219

choose dresses and suits that will make you appear thinner, but will you be able to stand up to their demands through an entire evening? If you purposely dress in clothes a size or two below your girth, make certain that the comfort you squeeze into is not momentary. You ladies know how embarrassing it can be for buttons to pop from your blouse into your soup; and many a man has told us how he spent a good part of his evening standing up just because he was afraid to tempt destiny (and the seat of his trousers) by sitting down too often. Why spoil an otherwise enjoyable evening by trying to force yourself to be something other than what you are? Eventually, if you follow our Plan, you may indeed become this person, but for now settle for being the individual that you are now. It is a lot more relaxing.

3. Consider, before your date, how you intend to treat your excess weight. Do you think it would be best to introduce it, or would it be better to ignore it? Your excess weight is like that third person crowding in where two's company. Do you just let it skulk about or do you bring it into the conversation? This is usually more of a consideration on a blind date, though first dates also can be laced with a certain trepidation even though the person you are dating has ostensibly seen what you look like. Whatever you do, don't try to joke your weight out of the picture. This is an obvious defense mechanism that will likely backfire, making your date feel uncomfortable and making you feel cheap. Your date is there because it is obviously you that he or she is interested in. Don't shift the emphasis to your weight. Making your weight the focus of the evening can mar whatever relationship you might be hoping for. The most extreme example we have heard of was told us recently by one of our young woman patients:

"I started to mention my diet," she said, "and it turned out that my date was also on it and we spent most of the evening talking about our weight problems. I can't remember his name but he's two hundred and forty-five pounds!"

Perhaps the best way to treat your overweight on a date is to accept it gracefully. If the subject should come up, your best response is: "Yes, I do have a weight problem but I'm taking care of

220

it," and shift the conversation to other ground. Keep your weight a very personal consideration. It really is just that.

4. Just because you are going out at night for dinner does not mean that you must starve yourself all day. In this instance you need not follow set eating times. You may want to use the "nibbler" diet we provide a bit later. We have found the menu listed below to be quite successful in taking you through the day as well as through your dinner date. It may happen that you are not hungry for dinner. In that case just order the minimum and, if you are hungry later, you can carry over the items you haven't eaten. *Be careful not to eat more.* If you have eaten all allowable items during dinner and your date runs into the early morning hours, you may select items to eat from Sunday's breakfast. Of course, you will have then utilized these foods and will not repeat them later Sunday morning. However, if your date has lasted this long, chances are that you will sleep through your Sunday breakfast time anyway.

Remember that your "total contentment" pill can be of great help today. It will allow you to eat less during the day so that you may save up your calorie expenditure for the evening. The last thing you want to do when you take someone out for dinner or are taken by someone is to sit at the table quietly turning away all the food. In such a case you'd be better off eating at home and dating after dinner This isn't nearly as much fun and we don't recommend it; after all, that is simply one more example of the "dietary imprisonment" that we don't want to put you through. Employ your "total contentment" pill to the maximum today and be extra certain you drink all your water *before* you go out for the evening. Not only will this prevent your forgetting about it during the course of the evening, but you will find that your hunger is far more controllable and you will be able to adhere more readily to the plan we've provided for you. So have a good time!

Your Dating Game Menu: Variation #1

Breakfast   ½ grapefruit OR 4 oz. orange juice
            coffee, tea
Lunch   Salad consisting of 4 oz. of the following: carrots, celery,

*radishes, mushrooms (raw), cucumber, lettuce, 3 slices
tomato and house dressing.
coffee, tea
You may nibble at this salad throughout the afternoon if
you wish, or you may eat it all at one sitting. You will get
more "wear" out of it if you stretch it out, we've found.*

Dinner *(eaten out)*

Appetizer: Your choice of the following: 4 oz. shrimp or crabmeat
cocktail or 1 doz. cherrystone clams or oysters

OR

Your choice of the following soups (8-oz. portions:) gazpacho,
minestrone, mushroom (not creamed), onion, pepper pot, tomato
or vegetable.

Salad: Your choice of 4 oz. of the following: tossed green,
spinach, any mixed green. (Standard "tossed" salad at many
restaurants may be three different lettuces with some sliced
radishes and/or mushrooms, perhaps with onion and celery. Any of
these combinations is fine.) Use a dressing of lemon juice or vinegar
and oil. Some restaurants provide a "diet" dressing. If you wish to
inquire about this you may do so, but our advice is to do so
discreetly; some maître d's take strong exception to this line of
questioning. If the restaurant where you are dining provides a salad
bar, your choice of ingredients is made even easier as you will be
mixing them yourself. Stick heavily to the greens, avoiding anchovies (they are salty and will add weight to you, if not fat) and the
various cheeses and bacon bits. Raw onion topping off a mixed
green salad is fine if you know your date pretty well, but you may
want to avoid it if it's the first time out. Watch out for the pickled
cucumbers; a little will go a long way because of the brine (salt) from
the pickling process.

Entree: You may have a good 6-oz. portion of any of the following:
striped bass, lobster, brook trout, flounder, scallops, haddock,
mussels.

Alcohol: You may have a 4-oz. glass of white wine with dinner or
a 1-oz. cocktail (not a mixed drink) before dinner. In either instance
you will not have dessert, but will finish the meal with coffee or tea.
An exception to this is that if you haven't finished your "must"

snack fruit for today—that is, the cranberries, strawberries, honeydew, watermelon or canteloupe—you may use one of these options for dessert and have the liquor as well. It is something to plan ahead for.

If you decide not to have the allowed quota of alcohol, you may stop there or you may choose from among the following fruits for dessert:

4 oz. applesauce, pineapple chunks, fruit cocktail
OR the following pastries:
4 Oreo cookies, ½ doughnut (plain), 2 fig bars, 2 macaroons,
2 chocolate wafers.

A couple of questions usually arise here. One woman asked: "How do I order half a doughnut?" (You see, we overweights never like to throw food away.) The answer is that you can't order half a doughnut; you only eat half. Put the remaining half on another plate; in a neutral corner, as it were. Then eat your half slowly, preferably breaking off small pieces for delicate bites with your coffee. The other question that usually comes up is: "How am I going to weigh out food at a restaurant? Surely, doctor, you don't expect me to carry my postage scale with me when I go out?"

No, of course we don't. However, we do expect you to be weighing items at home all during the course of the Nine-Day Plan, so by this time you should have a pretty good eye for what a six-ounce piece of fish or chicken or steak looks like, as well as approximately the volume taken up by four ounces of juice. Remember, we said "approximately." We don't expect you to be absolutely perfect. However, we do expect you to stop eating when this "approximate" quota of yours has been reached.

This may be a little difficult at first, since it may mean leaving food in excess of your quota on your plate. However, this is something you must learn to do. In some cases you can ask the waiter for a "small" portion and feel a little more psychologically secure; chances are you'll get the same size portion you'd have been served regardless. Don't eat it all just to please your date. Above all, don't worry about "wasting" food by letting it go back to the kitchen. You'll be wasting it more by adding it to the too much you are already carrying.

And, of course, you can always take the extra food home with you in a "doggie" bag. While this may pose some problems on a date, it is easy enough to do when out with your spouse. Many people who take home "doggie" bags haven't had a doggie in the house for years, if ever. There's no law saying you can't eat this food the following day; you've paid for it and there is no shame involved in bringing it home if it can possibly be managed. It may just help you cut down on what is left on your plate, since you know the food isn't going to be thrown away. For many people this is the most important factor of all.

AND FOR YOU MARRIEDS, A HEALTHIER RELATIONSHIP

Although so far we've been discussing going out on Saturday night more from a single's dating point of view, because we feel this viewpoint has been neglected, this doesn't mean that you marrieds can't utilize the same program. You would think that going out with your spouse would be easier than going out on a first date with a stranger, at least as far as your overweight is concerned. After all, your weight is nothing new; you don't have to try to overcome it; it isn't an intrusive factor in the relationship.

That's what you'd like to think.

Our experience has shown that overweight people are always conscious of their weight when out in public. Thus, even when you are dining out with your spouse you may feel your weight pointing a finger at you. This is not helped by having your dining partner constantly pointing a finger at you as well, telling you what you should or should not be eating. This is *your* job and yours alone. Whether or not to abide by any weight-loss program must be your decision. Conversely, your problem is certainly not helped by your spouse constantly telling you to eat just because you happen to be out for dinner. Our experience has shown us how often this happens. Once, a friend of ours, having just been released from the hospital and quite overweight, was out for dinner with his wife. She kept pushing on him all his favorite dishes—mostly heavy carbohydrates—because, as she said, "After what you've been through you deserve to pamper yourself." If you are the recipient of this sort of attention, you must be no less determined than your partner. Say: "Just a minute. That isn't on my diet. And my diet is what I must follow whether I am out for dinner or at home if I want to become that slimmer, more attractive and healthier individual I see waiting in the wings." And your spouse must understand this and be content with the fact that you are following, as in the Nine-Day Plan, a medically proven method for guaranteed weight loss that will make you this more desirable person. After all, you aren't imposing *your* diet on your spouse, so it is important that your spouse understand that he or she can't impose his or her diet on *you*. You've plenty to eat with the variations *we've* provided you to keep you full and contented through all of Saturday as well as Saturday night.

Marital Dining Out: Variation #2
Breakfast *½ cup cornflakes or Rice Krispies*
½ cup skim milk
coffee, tea
Lunch *4 oz. tomato juice*
1 egg, hard-boiled or fried in Teflon pan
6 asparagus spears, fresh or canned (may use in omelet)
coffee, tea
Dinner (out)
Soup: Your choice of black bean, borscht, chicken gumbo, cream of lobster, cream of mushroom, tomato soup with rice
OR
Alcohol (a predinner cocktail): 1 oz. whiskey, gin, rum or vodka
Entree: 4 oz. of any of the following: chicken, liver, kidney, rabbit, pheasant, swordfish, turkey (only light meat), veal. The chicken and turkey must be without skin. The liver may have fried onions with it.
Vegetable: 4 oz. of any two of the following: cauliflower, mushrooms, sauerkraut, spinach, squash, string beans
Beverage: coffee, tea

The Saturday Night Special: Variation #3
This one is for when you are really planning to make an evening of it, either for a special party of your own or in attending a wedding or other social event. In preparation for what you will eat this

evening you will not eat your special "must" foods today.

Breakfast *4 oz. tomato OR V-8 juice*
1 piece Melba toast
coffee, tea

Lunch *1 thin slice bread*
4 oz. cabbage
4 oz. green pepper
4 oz. cucumber } *mix into slaw with house dressing*
4 oz. celery
1 oz. onion
garlic

Dinner (out)

Alcohol variation (predinner cocktail): 1½ oz. whiskey, rum, gin, vodka

Appetizer: fruit cocktail, ½ grapefruit, 4 oz. tomato juice, ½ medium cantaloupe (choose 1)

Soup: any bouillon or beef or chicken broth

Entree: 4 oz. of beef, sausage, lamb or turkey (dark meat, skinned)

Vegetable: Choose any two: asparagus, broccoli, cabbage, spinach, mushrooms, string beans

Beverage: coffee or tea

Alcohol-Wine Variation

Start as above with the predinner cocktail, but skip the appetizer. You may substitute for this a two-ounce portion of any light table wine with your main course.

Preparation of the above foods is almost unlimited, provided you remember: a) no deep-fat fried foods, b) nothing breaded and c) nothing excessively rich, as in heavy cheeses or French sauces. Even here you can eat the food; just separate it from the overlying slush.

Nonalcoholic Variation

Why are so many people apologetic because they aren't having a predinner drink? It isn't mandatory, you know. Yet just the other day we had a patient tell us, "You know, I love your Nine-Day Plan, and I really do well on it during the week. But why do I have to drink all that alcohol on the weekends?"

Well, of course you don't have to drink any alcohol at all. Just because it is offered doesn't mean you must accept it. All the same, people who have rarely had a predinner cocktail seem to feel suddenly that they are missing something if they don't have one, since it is offered on their diet. Nonsense; you can have just as good a time without it because you can make up the extra calories on food. This kind of true eating will fill you up longer and give you more contentment than you would ever get from a drink you don't really want. Why, then, do we offer it? Because many people do want the comfort of that predinner cocktail; their choice of caloric expenditure includes that important purchase. If you'd just as soon do without the alcohol, the menu below might be more your style (again, you will not eat your "must" fruits today with this dinner):

Breakfast 4 oz. tomato OR V-8 juice
             1 piece Melba toast
             coffee, tea

Lunch 1 thin slice bread ⎫
          1 hard-boiled egg ⎪
          4 oz. lettuce   ⎬ as open sandwich
          1 slice tomato   ⎪
          coffee, tea   ⎭

Dinner
Appetizer: fruit cocktail, ½ grapefruit, 4 oz. tomato juice, ½ medium cantaloupe (choose 1)
Soup: any bouillon or beef or chicken broth
Entree: 5 oz. beef, sausage, frankfurter, lamb, dark-meat turkey, liverwurst or tongue
                        OR
4 oz. corned beef, duck (without skin), ham, pork, beef sweetbreads
Vegetable: 1 of the following: asparagus, broccoli, cabbage, spinach, mushrooms, string beans
Beverage: coffee, tea

The Saturday Night Extra-Special: Variation #4

This is for a truly special occasion when you want to celebrate with food and/or drink and still stay on your diet. You might even want

227

to use it to celebrate the successful termination of your first Nine-Day Cycle. That's one of the best excuses we know to celebrate, since even the celebration will be helping your weight loss.

As with the previous variation, you will not eat your "must" fruits for today with this one.

Breakfast ½ medium cantaloupe
  coffee, tea

Lunch 4 oz. tomato juice
  4 oz. celery, 4 oz. lettuce, 6 asparagus spears, 4 oz. green pepper, house dressing or lemon juice
  coffee, tea

Midafternoon (optional) 4 oz. either cranberries (do not use sauce) or strawberries

Dinner (out)

Alcohol variation (predinner drink): two 1-oz. drinks whiskey, gin, rum or vodka. These may be mixed with water, seltzer or diet soda. No other type of mixed drink is allowed.

Appetizer: fruit cocktail or ½ grapefruit

Soup: consommé (beef, chicken, oxtail), onion, mushroom (not creamed)

Entree: 8 oz. chicken breast (no skin) or brook trout

OR

6 oz. liver or veal

OR

4 oz. beef or lamb

Vegetable: Choose 1 of the following: spinach, cauliflower, sauerkraut, summer squash (4 oz.)

Beverage: coffee, tea

Alcohol-Wine Dinner Variation

In the above dinner, instead of the two 1-ounce highballs, drink only one and substitute for the second three ounces of a standard table wine (not a sweet one). If you decide that one drink is all you wish to have and you do not want any wine, do not substitute anything for the drink you aren't having. Don't drink alcohol just because it is allowed; don't drink two cocktails if you are satisfied with one; and don't drink even one if you are satisfied with none.

Alcohol-Wine-Brandy Variation

You may add one ounce of brandy to the above dinner by substituting it for the appetizer and the soup. If you wish *only* to have the brandy, eat the appetizer and soup but do not utilize the cocktails or the cocktail-wine combination. If you wish to start your meal with a cocktail and finish with brandy, this is also possible if you have only a single cocktail and no wine with the meal.

A Further Word About Alcohol

If, as is said, the proof of the pudding is in the eating, certainly the proof of the spirit is in the drinking. Any distilled spirit (such as whiskey, rum, vodka, gin) has a caloric content that depends on its proof—that is, the amount of alcohol that it contains. You can save yourself a lot of calories and still drink comfortably by imbibing lower-proof rather than higher-proof alcohol. You can specify what proof you want when you are out; certainly you can accommodate yourself this way when you are at home. Just to give you an example, a spirit of 150 proof (75 percent alcohol) will provide over 125 calories per fluid ounce, while the same spirit at 80 proof (40 percent alcohol) will furnish not quite 70 calories per ounce. This can be a saving to you of over 50 calories per drink—and you'll never notice the difference. We've started this habit for you by calculating all distilled spirits at 80 proof; be sure you make it a habit to order them this way.

The Nonalcoholic Dinner

We're still involved in that Saturday night extra-special occasion, but this time without any alcoholic drinks. The menu for the day stays the same, but the caloric allowance for alcohol will be turned back to you in the way of food as follows:

Appetizer: Your choice of fruit cocktail, ½ grapefruit, shrimp or crabmeat cocktail, mussels, oysters, clams (4 oz.)

Soup: Any of the soups in the previous menus for this evening

Entree: 8 oz. chicken (any part, with skin), salmon, swordfish, veal, turkey, mackerel, liver, lake trout, whitefish, shad roe, bluefish, rabbit

OR

6 oz. beef (all cuts if medium-fat), lamb, turkey (any portion, without skin), liverwurst

OR

4 oz. corned beef, duck, ham, pork (not fried, preferably grilled or broiled. Spare ribs are included here; you may use barbecue sauce).

Vegetable: 4 oz. of any 2: spinach, cauliflower, sauerkraut, summer squash, asparagus, broccoli, string beans

Beverage: coffee, tea

The Saturday Night Surprise Outing

You've been happily following your Nine-Day Wonder Diet all day. You've had breakfast and lunch according to the proper specifications; now it's four o'clock in the afternoon and your spouse, boy- or girlfriend calls and says, "I've just won a thousand dollars on the sweepstakes; let's celebrate by going out for dinner." Wonderful. However, you've not expected this so you've been following one of the basic menu variations for this day. You can't suddenly switch over to a "dining out" menu. If you do, you will be breaking one of the cardinal rules of the Nine-Day Plan: no switching from one menu to another. You will throw off the calculations we have made for your CBO time, and you will disrupt your diet. So what do you do?

There is only one thing to do, short of staying home, which would be ridiculous. Imagine saying to someone who has just given you this piece of good news, "I'm sorry, I can't go out. I'm on this diet that doesn't call for dining out today." No, go out. We want you to go. But you must take the remainder of your basic plan with you. Stay with the menu you've started. We will shortly be offering you a number of variations on the basic plan but you must, even here, stay with the particular variation you've chosen for the day. Remember, no matter what occasion arises, the occasion you are celebrating is constant, healthful weight loss. Never sacrifice this occasion to another; no matter how meatier it may look at a moment's notice, it has to prove, in the long run, much less fruitful. Haven't you proved this to yourself over and over again? Isn't it time to stop seeking excuses and to just plain succeed? Obviously it is, or you wouldn't have gotten this far in the Plan. Certainly one eating splurge isn't worth marring everything you've done to this point. So go out, but take your head along—the top part as well as the bottom part. And never let the bottom portion rule the top. That's how you got to be overweight to begin with. With the Nine-Day Wonder diet you can change all that, so you can finally lose your excess weight and never regain it. That, not excess eating, is the greatest thing you can do for yourself.

VARIATIONS ON TODAY'S BASIC MENU (AT-HOME PLAN)
Variation #1
Breakfast ½ cup orange juice
1 piece Melba toast
4 oz. skim milk
coffee, tea

Lunch ½ cup radishes
½ cup cucumbers
½ cup scallions
½ cup green pepper
2 tablespoons plain sour cream or yogurt
1 piece thin toast
coffee, tea

Dinner ½ grapefruit
4 oz. lobster (no butter sauce)
½ cup mushrooms
½ cup green pepper
3 slices tomato
coffee, tea

Variation #2
Breakfast ½ grapefruit
⅓ cup cottage cheese
1 piece Melba toast
coffee, tea

Lunch 1 cup skim milk or buttermilk
1 egg fried in Teflon pan

3 slices tomato
lemon juice
4 oz. lettuce
coffee, tea
Dinner 4 oz. broiled flounder
8 oz. spinach
6 stalks asparagus
coffee, tea

Variation #3
Breakfast 1 large biscuit shredded wheat
1 glass skim milk (8 oz.)
coffee, tea
Lunch ½ medium canteloupe
8 oz. vegetable soup
1 thin slice toast
coffee, tea
Dinner 4 oz. beef or chicken bouillon
4 oz. chicken breast (no skin)
1 small fresh ear of corn (or ½ cup canned, not creamed, corn)
coffee, tea

Variation #4
Breakfast ½ cup tomato juice
2 pieces Ry-Krisp
2 teaspoons jelly
coffee, tea
Lunch: 4 oz. water-packed canned tuna
4 oz. chopped onion
4 oz. chopped celery
coffee, tea
Dinner: 4 oz. broiled flounder
4 oz. broccoli
4 oz. cucumber
coffee, tea

Variation #5

Breakfast ⅔ cup Cream of Wheat
1 piece Ry-Krisp
1 teaspoon jelly
8 oz. skim milk or buttermilk
coffee, tea

Lunch 4 oz. shrimp cocktail (2 teaspoons sauce only)
4 oz. lettuce
8 oz. Campbell or Heinz Manhattan-style clam chowder
½ dozen oysterettes
coffee, tea

Dinner 4 oz. broiled striped bass
lemon juice
½ cup chopped onion
4 oz. green pepper
4 oz. cucumber
coffee, tea

EXCEPTIONAL RULES FOR TODAY

1. You may carry over calories from one meal to the next if you desire. This will help if you decide suddenly to go out to dinner and haven't eaten all your lunch selections. Or, if you skipped some of the breakfast portions, you make these up at lunch. We have calculated the CBO of these menus so you may do this readily. However, you may add only items from the previous meal to the next one; you may not, for instance, add uneaten foods from breakfast to the dinner menu.

2. Please do not eat items simply because they are allowed. We are trying to work with you because of the nature of the day. Don't work against yourself. Just the idea of dining out, or the ambience of a dinner party at home on a Saturday night in particular, is stimulating to many people's appetites. Remember, the calories you take in at the evening meal are the hardest for your body to get rid of; these are the incipient bumps and bulges of tomorrow. Keep that in mind as you swallow them down, and take them with caution for a seasoning.

233

3. All eating times today are variable. You may nibble all through the day if you wish, provided you do not eat more than the listed items. It's a good idea to write down the foods you eat so you won't eat them twice, either through thoughtless nibbling or from forgetting, when you carry a food over from one meal to the next, that you've already polished it off once. It is easy to forget. If you put your faith in your memory to remind you that you've already had your quota, you will find this a very sneaky guide. We urge all our patients to write down this Saturday's foods and drink. We repeat, this day is a critical juncture in the Plan. You can make or break, today, everything you've worked so hard for to this point. Take the few moments involved and write down what you are eating. And don't be like one of our patients, whose food list showed some items repeated three and four times. "I wrote everything down," she confessed, "but I was afraid to read the darn thing."

4. We said earlier that if you are going to be out this evening until early morning, you may utilize Sunday's breakfast items to fill in if you get hungry. This is the only instance in the entire cycle in which this is permitted, and we want to stress that you will not eat again on Sunday until the noon eating zone. As you will see, unlike Saturday, Sunday is a structured day as far as eating times are concerned.

Whether you go out Saturday night or stay home; whether you are married or single; whether you have only a few pounds to lose or many—you need not fear the weekend as far as the Nine-Day Wonder Diet is concerned. We almost want to say that you can just about forget that you are *on* a diet, but this is a risky boast to make. Remember that you *are* on a diet; just forget the notion that being on a diet has to be frustrating or uncomfortable or involve a total change of life-style. The only change you will be making in your life-style for the Nine-Day Plan is for the better in every way. Tomorrow is your last day of the cycle. You should have every reason to look forward to it as another, perhaps the last, step in the right direction.

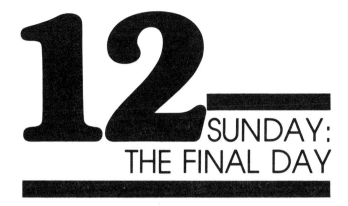

12

SUNDAY:
THE FINAL DAY

How you begin this last day of the Nine-Day Cycle depends, to some extent, on how you spent last night. If you were out late and impinged on this morning's breakfast, your eating day will start at noon. If you were either at home Saturday night, or did not eat beyond the items permitted, your Sunday eating will begin at breakfast time just as on any other day.

At the same time, we recognize that Sunday is not a day like any other, especially this Sunday, and we have attempted to accommodate some of the individual variations this day may bring.

SLEEPING IN

Sunday, for you, may be a late-rising day. You need not change this habit to suit the Nine-Day Plan; we have allowed for this possibility. Get up whenever you like; the rule of thumb here is that if you rise after ten in the morning but before noon, you may combine breakfast and lunch with the "brunch" menu. Of course, if you have eaten breakfast while out during the early morning hours, you will have to wait until the lunchtime zone to eat, though if you were wise and left a few items over, these leftover breakfast choices can carry you nicely until lunch. If you are one of those people who is fortunate enough to have his or her breakfast served in bed on Sunday, it might be wise for you to make copies of some of the menu choices for this day and pin them up where obliging members of your family can read them. It is embarrassing to be served breakfast in bed and have to turn down most, if not all, the food that is offered. A number of our patients have gotten into trouble this way. As one woman put it, "My husband and my little girl brought me breakfast in bed on Mother's Day. It consisted of all the foods I love but which, for the most part, weren't on the day's schedule. What was I going to do, make them feel bad by turning it away? I ate everything to make them happy."

How tragic and yet how human. And how avoidable, if only you notify your family just what foods are allowed you. Then, if they persist in bringing you "goodies" that aren't your cup of tea, you had better find out if they are really happy with your being fat; if so, you must make certain they realize that you aren't happy being that way. Breakfast in bed is fine; but the thoughtfulness that supplies that gesture ideally won't short-circuit itself halfway. If it does, you must not contribute to the confusion. Take what you can from the tray and turn back the rest with thanks. Next time, whoever brings you breakfast in bed will know that if it is really meant to please and surprise you, it will contain only those foods that will add to your pleasure for the day by keeping you on your diet.

GOING OUT SUNDAY NIGHT

You may go out for dinner Sunday night as well as Saturday night but you must stick to the menu you have chosen for the day. However, if you have not gone out Saturday night, and Sunday evening comes up strong for dinner out, you may utilize any of the Saturday Out-For-Dinner menus, including the alcohol. Remember, this is only the case if you've spent the previous evening using either the Basic Menu or one of the Variations. You may not use the "Saturday Night Special" on Sunday, for instance, if you've already used it on Saturday.

UNEXPECTED GUESTS

Sunday afternoon seems to be a good time for people just to drop in. If you run that sort of a house there is no reason for you to

236

live in a less free and easy style simply because you are dieting. You can entertain your guests and even have a drink with them on the "Drop-In" menu we have provided as one of the variations for today. Of course, you can always stick with the menu you started with and just have a cup of coffee with your guests; as we keep pointing out, alcohol is not mandatory. It depends on how you like to spend your Sunday. As for eating, if you are going to serve your guests so-called junk foods, such as potato chips, Fritos, pretzels, and such, you need not join them as another "junkie"; in the "Drop-In" menu we have given you more substantial things that you can nibble, socialize and still lose weight with.

And, of course, if you find that time goes by and you decide either to go out to eat with your guests or to serve them at home, the basic menu variations we have provided for today, together with your possibility of substituting last night's extra menus—if you haven't already used them—should take care of that with no difficulty. So, as you can see, the Nine-Day Wonder Diet prevents you from hitting those stumbling blocks that may have swerved you off all those other diets you've tried. We provide for just about every eventuality. In the years we've been working in the field of weight reduction we've heard just about every difficulty, every temptation that can arise to make you go off your Plan. We can't avoid them for you, but we can show that there are planned alternatives to them so that you are never at a loss as to what to do. Your choices are clearly defined. Our own experiences, when we were fat, have shown us that trouble with going off one's diet usually arises when one is trying to cope with an unforeseen situation. In the Nine-Day Plan, as little as possible is left unforeseen.

EXPECTED GUESTS

Sunday is also a day for planned visits from family and friends. Here you may be preparing for a large dinner or a small, more intimate one. There is still no need for you to go off your diet. What you will be doing is incorporating all the foods that you can eat into the meal in general. Then, while dining, you will simply pull these ingredients back out. No one need know—and, especially if the guests are family, no one *should* know—that you are dieting.

Relatives can be very cruel. We have never been able to figure out the pleasure some people get from actually taunting others with food. One of our patients came to us in tears telling us how her relatives had made fun of her, rather viciously, for sticking to her diet in the midst of a family dinner. "I made the mistake of telling them what I was doing," she said, "and I paid the price in taunting and ridicule. But the more fun they made of me, the more determined I became to stick to it. And I did. And all I could think of was, 'I'll be thin when you're still fat.' "

One major caution with expected guests. If you are the cook, don't experiment with entirely new recipes when you are on the Nine-Day Plan. You know that you are going to have to taste, sometimes quite extensively, the mixtures that you will be blending to make sure the ingredients are quite right. Any good cook (and we pride ourselves in being two good ones) *has* to taste as he or she goes along when making something entirely new. We all want to impress our guests with what good cooks we are—but impress them with something tried and true; don't go out on a limb with something new. If you do, the necessity to taste as you go along won't do your limbs a bit of good; they'll get heavier as you continue to absorb the extra calories that aren't on your Plan and that will stifle the fires of your CBO.

"I don't understand why I didn't lose more weight," one man told us. "I stuck to the Plan all nine days... well, except for Sunday. I like to cook and I had these guests I especially wanted to impress so I whipped up a really great recipe I'd been given. But I didn't eat any of it." We asked him if he'd tasted as he went along. "Well, of course, I *tasted*," he admitted. "I couldn't be sure it was coming out right otherwise. Do you mean *that* could have done it? Just that little bit?" Yes, we do mean exactly that. That little bit can do in your entire Plan. It may be hard to conceive this but consider, if you will, how small a bullet is. All the same, it can kill you. What you may consider just a little bit of food can do the same to your diet. Don't taste, even if you are going to spit it out. First of all, most people can't spit it out. Once it is in their mouth it is good for the entire trip. And, even if you are one of those rare individuals who can spit it out, you will still absorb a good deal of this unwanted food through the mucous membranes of the mouth. Better to use a recipe that you've used many times before, that you know will work according to proven proportions and that you don't have to taste, than one that's new and that you have to keep checking on.

Of course there are cooks who have to keep tasting everything no matter how many times they've made it before. They do this almost by reflex. To you we say, get out of the habit. Remember how often you've produced this dish to the applause of your guests. You've the proper proportions all ready, at your fingertips; you certainly don't need them in your mouth as well. Stop tasting. And stop worrying about whether the dish will work as well if you don't taste. Believe us, it will. You are just using another excuse to eat; it is the same habit pattern that helped get you fat. It is part of the habit pattern that you will have to change in order to get thin and stay that way. It really isn't hard to break the pattern; all you must do is remember that cooking and eating are two different activities altogether, not part of the same general grouping. Once you have that firmly fixed in your mind before you start cooking, you will have no trouble. We, ourselves, cook at times for large groups of people. We then sit and eat with them, but if we are back on the Nine-Day Plan because we've gained a few pounds, we don't eat *for* them. We don't taste as we are preparing the food (we already know what it tastes like), and when we sit down to eat we accumulate on our plates only those foods that are permitted for that day. In this fashion both of us lost our weight many years ago and in this fashion we have both stayed at our normal weight to this day.

IF YOU ARE VISITING

On any particular Sunday, including this one, instead of staying at home receiving visitors, you may be doing the visiting. Obviously, when you are in someone else's house you haven't the control of the food that is possible to you at home. But this doesn't mean that you must put yourself entirely at the mercy of the household you happen to be visiting. You can pick and choose among the items offered, selecting those that are on this day's menu from among those that aren't. And you can do this without offending the host or hostess, without making a big fuss about being on a diet. In fact, you shouldn't mention to your hosts that you are dieting at all. If anyone asks why you are not eating a particular item, lie. Say that you are on a restricted food intake because of an ulcer or hemorrhoids. Or just use the old line about being "allergic" to this particular food. You'll be surprised how readily this excuse will be accepted. Meanwhile you will most likely have found plenty to eat that is on your Plan, so that you won't have to go home hating yourself and dreading the fact that tomorrow, Monday, you will be weighing yourself and all those extra calories will be waving to you from the scale.

As far as your water drinking is concerned, we suggest that if you are tempted to eat at someone else's house, you drink a couple of extra glasses of cold water instead. Everyone has water available, and this is one item you can partake of at will. Certainly there is no excuse for *not* drinking your water just because you are out. It's funny the ideas some people have about water, associating it strictly with their own kitchen tap. "I couldn't drink all my water yesterday because I was visiting," one patient told us. When we asked if the home she was visiting was equipped with plumbing she admitted it was. "But I never thought of drinking my water there. They'd have thought I was crazy."

If you feel self-conscious, go into the bathroom and pour yourself some water from the tap there. Some people won't drink water from a bathroom tap, considering it "different" from the water they get from the kitchen tap. It's the same water. And it's the same water you get at any home you happen to be visiting. So don't worry about drinking it. Let your hosts know you like it. As one of our patients said, raising his glass of water, "My compliments to the chef." He told us, "My hosts were delighted with the remark. It showed them I appreciated their home. It also took their attention away from a lot of the foods they were serving that I couldn't eat, as they weren't on my day's menu."

People you are visiting like to hear compliments about their home. After all, this is the hub of their hospitality. They associate the food they are serving with this same hospitality. Make yourself as agreeable as possible about the house, the grounds, the pictures on the walls. But as far as the food is concerned, what isn't on your

240

day's Plan you must draw the line at. Otherwise that line will become a rope around your neck.

It may happen to you, as it has to a few of our patients, that on some rare occasion you find yourself visiting at a home where there is absolutely nothing to eat that is on your Plan. The logical thing to do here is go home hungry and satisfy yourself with our special "frustration" dinner. We have arranged this specifically for such an occasion. What do you say to your hosts on this occurrence? The best idea could be to plead ill and escape the precincts as soon as possible. If, food aside, you are having a good time and don't want to leave, you can always say that you were confused about whether or not they were having dinner and ate earlier. It is, admittedly, an awkward situation, but not nearly so awkward for you as if you eat simply to get out of it. That way you will carry around with you an even more awkward situation. But don't be ashamed about making excuses *not* to eat. You will, very likely, find it a fascinating change of pace. And you will be surprised to find how willing people are to believe whatever you say about your relationship to food provided you don't tell them the real reason: that you are not eating because you will get fatter if you do. That seems to be the one excuse that no host or hostess will put up with.

WHAT YOU WILL EAT TODAY

1. Eight 8-ounce glasses of cold water divided through the day and one extra 8-ounce glass of water at bedtime. That's right, today there will be nine glasses in all. You should have no trouble getting the extra glass down, with all the experience drinking water that the past eight days have provided. Today being the ninth day, we celebrate with nine glasses of water. If we can do it, you can do it. In fact, on some days, we drink over ten glasses of water, spread throughout our waking hours. Water is the best weight-reduction medicine there is.

2. Your multivitamin-mineral tablet.

3. If you have been taking your "total contentment" pill, be sure you continue it through today. This will be the last day that you will be using these items for a crutch. As we keep pointing out, they won't do the job for you but they will certainly make it easier for you to do the job.

241

4. Tea and/or coffee, as much as you want, with one teaspoon of whole milk or nondairy creamer as you wish. You may, of course, drink it black. You may, as usual, have lemon in your tea.

5. Have 4 oz. of either tomato juice or grapefruit or orange sections, unsweetened (we prefer Kraft, fresh, dairy-packed, but come as close as you can to these) at noon, 4 P.M. and 8 P.M. You have a half-hour variation here; if you miss these times by more than a half hour either way, skip that portion. You may alternate the items or stick solely to one; the choice is yours. We would like you, as usual, to drink the juice as slowly as possible, sitting down. If you choose to eat the sections they, like anything you eat, must be chewed well and never while standing.

6. You may have up to three cans of diet soda today at any time of the day you wish. Remember, neither the diet soda nor the coffee or tea takes the place of the water you will drink.

EATING TIMES FOR TODAY (BASIC TIME ZONES)

Breakfast: From 8 A.M. to 10 A.M.
Brunch (optional; if you miss breakfast *only*): 10 A.M. to noon
Lunch: 12 noon to 1 P.M.
Dinner: 3 P.M. to 6 P.M.

You must eat nothing after 6 P.M. on the basic Plan or on any of the alternates unless it is so specified. Your next meal will be breakfast on Monday morning, after you have weighed yourself for the third and final time on the Cycle. If you miss any of the eating zones you cannot make up the skipped meal; the only exception is brunch, which will allow you to combine any two breakfast items with one lunch item, or vice versa. If you eat brunch at 10 A.M., that means you will not be eating again, until 3 P.M. at the earliest, so this eating time should be carefully considered. Brunch is supplied solely because of the possibility of your sleeping later on a Sunday morning.

BASIC MENU: DAY 9

Breakfast ½ *grapefruit*
 2 pieces Melba toast
 coffee, tea

Lunch *Caesar salad as follows: lemon juice, 4 oz. romaine lettuce; 1 egg, hard-boiled; 4 oz. green pepper; 4 oz. mushrooms; 4 oz. Boston lettuce, house dressing*
coffee, tea

Dinner *4 oz. breast of chicken*
6 fresh or canned asparagus stalks
4 oz. spinach
½ medium potato
coffee, tea

VARIATIONS ON THE BASIC MENU FOR THIS DAY
Variation #1
Breakfast *⅔ cup cornflakes or Rice Krispies*
8 oz. (1 cup) skim milk

Lunch *1 fried egg (use Teflon pan)*
6 stalks asparagus (fresh or canned)
1 piece Ry-Krisp
coffee, tea

Dinner *4 oz. broiled striped bass or brook trout*
4 oz. cabbage
4 oz. string beans
coffee, tea

Variation #2
Breakfast *1 egg, poached or fried*
1 piece Melba toast
1 teaspoon jelly
coffee, tea

Lunch *4 oz. shrimp*
4 oz. lettuce
4 oz. celery
4 oz. chopped onion
4 oz. green pepper
coffee, tea

Dinner *4 oz. lobster*   *3 slices tomato*
4 oz. sauerkraut   *coffee, tea*
4 oz. broccoli

Variation #3
Breakfast *4-oz. dish strawberries*
1 glass skim milk
coffee, tea
Lunch *8 oz. Campbell's vegetable soup with beef*
6 oysterettes
coffee, tea
Dinner *4 oz. veal*
4 oz. carrots
4 oz. cauliflower
coffee, tea

Variation #4
Breakfast *½ medium cantaloupe*
1 egg, boiled or poached
1 piece Melba toast
coffee, tea
Lunch *salad consisting of: 4 oz. raw spinach, 4 oz. shredded iceberg lettuce, 1 teaspoon diced onion, 1 teaspoon green pepper, 1 teaspoon pimiento, 4 oz. chopped orange slices, 4 oz. chopped cucumber, house dressing or lemon juice. Use salt substitute and pepper to taste.*
Dinner *1 cup of beef, chicken or vegetable bouillon*
4 oz. turkey (light meat only)
4 oz. cranberries
coffee, tea

Variation #5
Breakfast *4 oz. applesauce*
coffee, tea
Lunch *1 cup Manhattan-style clam chowder*
1 dozen cherrystone clams (raw) with horseradish
6 oysterettes
coffee, tea

Dinner *Vegetable dish consisting of: 1 small ear fresh or canned corn; fresh or canned beets; green pepper; string beans; lettuce and fresh cauliflower (4 oz. of each). coffee, tea*

Special Variation: Nibbling Food Instead of Junk Food

When everyone else is munching crackers, potato chips, pretzels or whatever, have the following available for yourself if you want to join in:

4 oz. raw carrot cut into long strips
4 oz. celery cut into long strips, after scraping
½ dozen green stuffed olives
½ dozen green olives with pits

Start your munching at the bottom of the list with the green olives with pits. Take your time nibbling the meat away from the pit. Use the pit as a pacifier; roll it around your mouth; get the most oral satisfaction you can from it before disposing of it. Next, you may want to go to the stuffed olives. Take one of these. Chew it up slowly. Remember that all this time you are talking, walking around the room, making sure your guests are comfortable. It isn't necessary for you to eat all the hors-d'oeuvres provided above; try to stay with the minimum. Next, perhaps you would like to attempt a piece of raw celery; you may use salt substitute with it. Last, try a piece of raw carrot. Ounce for ounce carrot has more calories than the other items, so use caution here. If, as happens, you forget in the heat of discussion and camaraderie that you must watch how often your hand moves to your mouth, and you look down and find that you've eaten all *your* particular "social foods," you may not have any more.

Whether you eat only part or all of these special nibbling foods, dinner that night must be that of Basic Variation #1, regardless which menu breakfast and lunch came from, or whether you ate breakfast or lunch at all. We have calculated this particular dinner to be best suited for the addition of such "nibbling" foods without a substantial loss of your CBO.

You will note that in permitting this, we have broken a rule that has been steadfast throughout the rest of the Plan. This has been: Never mix one menu with another. However, we have changed this rule a little for this day to give you the most social freedom possible. That doesn't mean you may now substitute and change menus at will. The rule of not mixing one menu with another still holds good except for such specific circumstances we may indicate as we go along.

Special Variation #2:
The "Drop-In" Menu

If you want to do more than just nibble along with your guests—if you want to join them in a drink, for instance—we have provided a way for you to do this and still not lose out on the demands of your diet. You may have one drink of distilled spirits: whiskey, gin, vodka or rum, provided it is no more than an ounce and provided you then eat for dinner no more than 4 oz. of any lean fish such as bass, haddock or flounder, together with no more than 4 oz. of a vegetable such as broccoli, cabbage, cauliflower or green pepper—*and nothing else.* If you haven't got these items in the house at the moment, and you don't see your way clear to getting them, better not have that drink.

Special Variation #3: Special Breakfast
for Late-Nighters

For those of you who are nightowls and get hungry in the wee hours, here's a breakfast variation you may utilize a little earlier than the rest of us—that is, provided you are still going fairly strong after midnight on Saturday and it looks as if you will need a bit more fuel to enjoy the rest of your time out. We've somewhat tipped the balance of the meals in favor of breakfast, but that doesn't mean this particular menu isn't available to anyone who wants to start off Sunday morning with a fairly substantial repast:

Breakfast ½ *cantaloupe*
1 five-inch strip bacon
1 fried egg
1 thin slice toast
coffee, tea

Lunch *1 cup clear beef or chicken bouillon*
Salad consisting of 4 oz. lettuce, 4 oz. fresh mushrooms, 4 oz. green pepper, 4 oz. celery. Lemon juice dressing.
coffee, tea

Dinner *4 oz. either liver or swordfish steak or veal*
4 oz. mushrooms or onion fried in Teflon pan
coffee, tea

Incidentally, a good brunch menu may be had by mixing any two of the above breakfast items with one from the lunch menu, or vice versa. You may prefer to have brunch rather than an early breakfast this day. It's up to you.

Special Variation #4: The Frustration Dinner

We promised that we'd let you get even if you managed to restrain yourself when you were out and could get nothing to eat that was on your Plan for the day. Since we cannot conceive this happening except on very rare occasions, you may have the following for dinner regardless what you've eaten for breakfast and lunch (provided, of course, that you have followed one of the listed menus for these meals):

½ grapefruit
3 oz. hamburger
slice of raw onion (or Teflon pan-fried)
4 oz. watermelon or ½ medium cantaloupe

LOOKING BACK ON NINE SUCCESSFUL DAYS

Now that you've come this far, actually having completed your first cycle on the plan, wasn't it worth it to stick to it? How could you have had any doubts? There was no question of staying on your diet and "starving" yourself. You ate at the proper times and you ate well. Being tempted to go off your diet—isn't that nonsense? Shouldn't the temptation rather work the other way, to make you want to stay on it, especially when, as with the Nine-Day Plan, the rewards are so great and the method so easy and comfortable?

Shakespeare said, "To thine own self be true," and this couldn't be a more apt proposal concerning your diet, if being thin is really what you want. If you want to be fat, certainly this is your choice as well. But if you've come this far, you must want to be thin—and you know by now there's no reason in the world you can't be. Certainly the past nine days have proved this to you. If you've more weight to lose, the next Nine-Day Cycle will show you even more clearly how fast you will be able to travel down the path toward a future that once seemed so far away. That particular future is, quite literally, in your hands. We have put into your hands a tool that will help you make this future a reality. Our promise to you is that it works. Your promise to yourself must be to use it.

13

ADDITIONAL VARIATIONS FOR SPEEDY WEIGHT LOSS

A lot, of course, depends on how much weight you have to lose. If you are only twelve pounds or less overweight, you may lose this in one cycle on the Nine-Day Plan. Unfortunately, most of the people we deal with in our practice have considerably more than this to lose. In such instances, we first place them on our Food Intake Plan as outlined in our book *You Can Be Fat-Free Forever,* which was designed for people at least twenty pounds over their normal weight. We vary this with either the basic Nine-Day Plan or some variation thereof.

This does not mean you can't lose a considerable amount of weight on the Nine-Day Plan alone. It is for this reason, calculating that most people will need more than one cycle, that we have spent a good deal of time figuring out the CBO for a great variety of menus. Before going on any of the variations discussed in this chapter you should have gone through the basic cycle, as discussed in the past chapters, at least once. After that, each additional cycle is up to you: you may combine the Basic Plan with one of these variations, or simply remain on the Basic Plan with the choices of menu you have there. If you are a particularly stubborn case, if you get bored easily, if you want even faster weight loss than you are getting after a cycle or two on the Basic Plan (and, needless to say, if you were following instructions while on it), you may find that the variations in this chapter will lose weight for you, as an individual with individual problems, even faster and more efficiently than did the Basic Plan alone.

INCREASING THE FAST DAYS

For some people fasting is so easy that they would rather not eat for three or four days straight than put food in their mouth to restimulate their hunger cycle. We have found that such fasting will increase the amount of weight you can lose on the Nine-Day Plan, but we do *not* advise that you undertake any prolonged fasting—that is, fasting for more than the two days in the Basic Plan—without getting an OK from your doctor. We believe you should have his permission even for fasting the two days, though we know the majority of people will do this on their own. Certainly if you think you can get through four or five days of eating nothing at all, it could be a worthwhile attempt. More than five days of fasting we definitely do not advise. Chances are that you would then be losing more "lean muscle mass"—that is, necessary body protein—than fat, and even if you were to take some sort of supplement, you could run into trouble unless you were being checked *every day* by a doctor. Our own experiences with prolonged weight-loss fasts have concerned patients who have been hospitalized specifically for this purpose—and almost all of these individuals regained all their weight once the fasting period was over.

So fasting, by itself, is really not enough, and most people wouldn't care to try an extended fast anyway. But fasting for three to five consecutive days can get the pounds off you rapidly. We suggest if you want to try it, that you start your fast on Monday and carry it through to Friday night, if you can last that long. For some people, making the length of their fast a specific goal stimulates the activity to continue; for others, such regimentation might only prove a stumbling block. We have found it best to fast "as we go along," taking the time as it comes, day by day...hour by hour, if need be. Follow the rules laid down in the chapters on fasting as to what to drink. Be certain, no matter how short or long your fast, that you take enough water, that you are aware of possible side effects as we have noted them, and that you take your multivitamin-mineral combination. You might also want your "total contentment" pill to help you along.

INTERSPERSING THE FAST DAYS

You may find it more convenient *not* to fast for two days straight. If so, you may break up the fast days, placing the first on Monday, the second on Wednesday and transposing Wednesday's Plan to Tuesday. If this works well for you and you wish to add a third fast day, incorporate this on Friday and simply cancel out the Friday Plan. We do not suggest that you fast on weekends. With the best will in the world, we feel (and experience has shown us to be right) that a weekend fast gets to be considered "punishment." If, despite our doubts on this score, you want to fast on a weekend, you may certainly do so. Of the two weekends involved in the Cycle, the second would probably be the best. We have had individuals plunge right into a weekend fast, introducing themselves to the Cycle that way, but we have found that most people wouldn't care for this.

PARTIAL FASTING FOR MORE THAN TWO DAYS

You may not be able to fast completely at all but partial fasting, as described in the chapters on fasting, may be just fine for you. You may want to continue this for another day or even two, rather than utilize the food days coming up. It is perfectly all right for you to try this for a cycle or two. We have had patients who even combined partial fasting will full fasting, using the two fast days to eat nothing at all, and the next two days to combine the food lists given for partial fasting rather than use the menus for those days. You may, if you wish, take the lists of permitted items for the partial fasting days and use these foods throughout the five weekdays of the Plan. We have purposely provided the caloric equivalents here so that you may, in effect, plan your own dieting control. This variation has worked wonders for many of our patients, but this must be *your* idea and you must remember that you are not bound to it. You may get off it any time and switch immediately to the foods offered for that particular day.

SUBSTITUTING FOOD DAYS

You may find that one food day works better for you than another. For instance, you may prefer two Fish and Fowl Days or two Full Protein Days rather than one of each. You may even prefer to eat nothing but Vegetables, Fruits and Dairy as we have provided them in that day for all five weekdays. You can lose weight doing this. We suggest that you combine at least one fast day with it, but we have had patients, particularly vegetarians, who have utilized the foods on this one day for all nine days and lost a lot of weight. If it is your choice to employ any one eating day for the entire Cycle or any part thereof, you will find enough variety in the menus provided to enable you to do so. That is one reason we have spent so much time giving you as much variety as possible. Variety is a funny thing; many people might find the idea of eating nothing but vegetables, or even vegetables, fruit and dairy, for nine days monotonous, not varied. It all comes down to what *you* want, how *you* like to eat. We've provided a way for *you* to eat what you like and still lose weight.

STARTING THE PLAN ON A DIFFERENT DAY

We have suggested that you begin your Nine-Day Wonder Diet on a Saturday and finish on the following Sunday, but it may not be convenient for you to do this. Our experience has shown that the day on which they start a Cycle makes a great deal of difference to most people's weight loss. Saturday is undoubtedly the best. If offers the most efficient psychological approach and our entire Plan is really based on a Saturday beginning. We strongly urge you to start just that way. However, if for some reason this would be extremely difficult and unwieldy for you to do, you can start with whatever day is available and go on from there—but you must always end the Cycle on a Sunday night even if you have to carry over three or four additional days to do it. It is certainly more awkward to do it this way, but if you don't, chances are your weight loss will not be what it should and everything will start getting rather slipshod. We have found that one difficulty with this Plan is to. get people to wait to start it. We may discuss it with a patient on Monday, for instance, and that person will be all on fire to start the

Plan the very next day. We always advise waiting until the proper day to start—Saturday; if you do this your chances of success in losing the weight you should are greatly increased.

THE "MONOTONY" CYCLE

With some people giving them any sort of choice so far as food is concerned is enough to stimulate them to eat everything in sight. If variety alone makes you hungry, we suggest that you try a specific, monotonous way of eating for several days. Take the lunch from the Basic Menu for Day 5, for instance, and apply that to each meal for four or even five days, as follows:

½ grapefruit
4 oz. beef broiled, grilled, pan-fried, baked. Beef should be lean.
seasoning to taste from zero-calorie list
4 oz. lettuce
4 oz. green pepper
coffee, tea

You can lose weight quite speedily here for two reasons. First, there are not other choices to make you hungry; second, by making your eating monotonous you are de-emphasizing its importance—thus, you will eventually pay less attention to it. It may sound incredible, but this is exactly what happens; we've proved it in our office with our patients many times. Of course, this doesn't happen immediately, but it will occur sooner than you might think. Give it a try, especially if you think there is too much food being offered you on the Nine-Day Plan.

The "Nibbler's" Variation

You may substitute this for any day when you feel you just can't stay on a structured plan that insists on specific eating "zones." It may be that you will be involved in activities this day that simply will not allow "structured" eating; you may, for instance, be spending the day in the hospital visiting someone who is quite ill. Your eating will be done in spurts, probably in the hospital luncheonette. There is no chance of controlling your eating times when you are in such emotional distress. Rather than have you feel guilty about "cheating" on your diet, try eating the following through the day:

253

Morning ½ grapefruit
toast (1 piece thin bread)
1 teaspoon jelly
coffee, tea

Afternoon 4 oz. hamburger without the bun, or any beef
slice raw onion
small portion lettuce and tomato salad
lemon dressing
coffee, tea

Evening 8 oz. preferably clear soup, or 8 oz. vegetable soup
4 oz. broiled fish (flounder, haddock, bass, scallops)
lemon juice
4 oz. cauliflower or broccoli
coffee, tea

The above items can be eaten in any order, singly or combined, at any time through the day. You do *not* have to eat them all. Be careful, if you are under stress at this time, that you don't eat just because you are nervous. It would be better for you to keep your jaws busy chewing gum, if, as it does with many people, moving your jaws proves a pacifier for you. But it is *only* your jaws that need pacifying—not your stomach.

The "Skipping Meals" Variation

We have gone to some pains to tell you, during the eating days, that if you skip a particular meal's time zone, you skip the meal. This is not meant to threaten you; it is, in fact, a good idea to skip meals if you are not hungry. Never eat just because "it's the time" to eat. We have had a great many people lose weight rapidly by skipping one or even two meals each day. There's nothing wrong with this, despite the fact that we were all brought up to believe we'd drop dead if we missed a meal. We've found only success and a clear conscience in people who miss as many meals as they can. The trick, of course, is to avoid the trap of skipping breakfast and lunch, say, and then feeling so virtuous about it that you eat twice as much for dinner as is on your Plan. Don't think, "Look how good I've been all day; don't I deserve a little extra something?" That little extra something you will gain by skipping meals where you can is

254

your stomach shrinking so that you will be hungry less often and require less food to be comfortable. It doesn't matter which meals you skip. You can eat breakfast and not eat till dinner, or not until the following day. As we keep reminding you, your face may not be eating but your body is. Your body is eating your fat—last week's breakfast, last week's lunch. Why add more to the stock if you don't need it? It's a good idea to carry with you not only while you are on the Nine-Day Plan, but for the rest of your life.

14

MAINTAINING YOUR WEIGHT LOSS: THE CYCLE-BALANCING PLAN

You've now completed your first Nine-Day Cycle; where do you go from here? A lot depends on how much more weight you have to lose. If one Cycle has just about gotten you down to where you should be, you are ready to go on our Maintenance Plan. You will stay on this Plan for at least two weeks, perhaps a month. During this time you will bring to bear on your eating habits all the things we have tried to get you to do while on the Nine-Day Plan. This change in your eating habits, called Behavior Modification, is necessary to prevent you from gaining back the weight that you have lost—from ever being fat again. It is discussed at great length in our previous book, *You Can Be Fat-Free Forever,* and we would recommend that you get a copy and follow the directions laid out in those pages. Once you have completed Maintenance and have your new eating pattern under control, you should then be able to return to eating "normally" along the caloric limits you have calculated for yourself. The basic Maintenance Plan you will follow if one cycle has taken you to normal weight goes like this:

Breakfast *4 oz. orange juice OR ½ grapefruit*

½ slice whole-wheat or rye toast with ½ teaspoon margarine

1 egg cooked hard or soft or fried in a Teflon pan
coffee or tea, no sugar, little milk (you may use a sugar
substitute)

Lunch *4 oz. tomato, V-8 or grapefruit juice*
6 oz. meat, fish or shellfish equivalent
2 tablespoons green or yellow vegetable
OR
lettuce and tomato
coffee, tea as above

Dinner *4 oz. tomato juice or its caloric equal*
1 cup bouillon (salt-free)
6 oz. meat, poultry, fish or shellfish equivalent
OR
2 eggs
1 small tossed salad with a low-calorie dressing

Dessert *Note: choice of one (1) only:*
¼ melon or 1 apple or 1 pear or 12 grapes or 6 oz. of any
stewed, water-packed fruit or 6 oz. of fresh berries or 1
small ball of ice milk or sherbet
coffee, tea as above

Remember: You will now be off the Nine-Day Plan and more or less on your own. At the end of each week you will weigh yourself. If you have gained weight, either you haven't stayed on your Maintenance Plan or you must cut down on some of the allowed items. It is never necessary to eat everything on the Maintenance Plan; eat as little as you can to remain comfortably full and satisfied. Eat slowly and chew well; the stomach has no teeth or taste buds. Avoid snacks except for one carrot and two stalks of celery, if you wish them, between meals. On weekends you may add half a dozen green olives (with pits) as a snack between meals. We would prefer you to have no alcohol at all while you are on the Maintenance Menu. This is to allow your CBO to stabilize; don't worry, you will get your alcohol back just as soon as you are on Control (see *Fat Free Forever*). Do not eat any white bread or rolls. Above all, don't stop drinking your water. The 8 eight-ounce glasses a day is to become a lifetime habit. Remember to keep your salt intake low, learn to use freshly ground pepper.

BALANCING YOUR INTAKE BETWEEN CYCLES

For many of you reading this book, one Cycle, even if it takes twelve pounds off you—more than a pound a day—will still leave you with a lot of weight to lose. When you complete a Cycle, we do not advise you to go on another immediately. You will be finishing your Cycle on Sunday at midnight. You cannot start another Cycle until the following Saturday. What do you do in the meantime, and how do you eat?

1. We suggest that you go on the Food Intake Plan from our previous book, *You Can Be Fat-Free Forever,* during the days between one Nine-Day Cycle and the next. This is a nonstructured, high-protein, low-carbohydrate plan that we use by itself to treat many of our excessively overweight patients. Not only will this plan carry you easily over the time between cycles, but in itself it will provide you with more weight loss and further information on Behavior Modification that will help you keep off what you lose.

2. At the same time, the Nine-Day Plan is, of itself, a complete entity and you can utilize it not only to lose weight, but to maintain (balance out) the weight you have lost while you are waiting for another Cycle to begin. This is the Cycle-Balancing portion of the Wonder Diet and it works as follows:

During any period between Cycles (it doesn't matter how long), you can maintain your weight by utilizing the menu lists provided during the eating days (there is no fasting during the period of Cycle Balancing) and combining them in various ways. For instance, you may take a breakfast from one menu, combine it with lunch from another from a different day, and do the same for your dinner choice. In other words, what you will be doing is just what we told you NOT to do when you were on the plan to lose weight. And that's why we told you not to do it; you'd be balancing yourself out. It is not by accident that this occurs; we planned it that way in order for you to have a complete, working entity at your disposal, for your disposal capabilities. It works just fine. Give it a chance to work for you.

A FINAL WORD

For some reason many people do not listen to instructions.

258

Perhaps they don't hear them, being too busy preparing themselves to ask another question. We have attempted, within the scope of this book, to provide for you a quick, surefire method to lose weight, one that you can follow without any bizarre circumstances in attendance. This Plan does not work by mumbo jumbo, by tearing you apart or by invoking your subconscious. If anything, what we want to invoke is your conscious. We want you to think. Thinking means following instructions. If you will do just that much, your Nine-Day Wonder Diet will do all the rest.

INDEX

274

275